Guinea Fowl : Genetics & Breeding

Guinea Fowl : Genetics & Breeding

Editors :

DEEPAK SHARMA, Ph.D.

Principal Scientist and Head

Division of Animal Genetics, Indian Veterinary Research Institute, Izatnagar-243 122 (U.P.)

HARPREET SINGH, Ph.D.

Principal Scientist (Rt)

Avian Genetics & Breeding, Central Avian Research Institute, Izatnagar 243 122 (U.P.)

SSPH

SATISH SERIAL PUBLISHING HOUSE

403, Express Tower, Commercial Complex
Azadpur, Delhi-110033 (India)
Phone : 011-27672852, Fax : 91-11-27672046
E-mail : info@satishserial.com,
hkjain1975@yahoo.com
Website : www.satishserial.com

Published by :

SATISH SERIAL PUBLISHING HOUSE

403, Express Tower, Commercial Complex, Azadpur,
Delhi-110033 (INDIA)
Phone : 011-27672852 Fax : 91-11-27672046
E-mail : info@satishserial.com,
hkjain1975@yahoo.com

ISBN 978-93-81226-48-3

Typeset at: Harminder Kharb *for* Laxmi Art Creation
Printed at: Salasar Imaging Systems, Delhi-110035

Contents

Preface

Poultry farming is recognized as a potential tool to fight poverty and malnutrition with tremendous employment opportunity. In India, poultry production has increased rapidly and tremendously in the last three decades, but this expansion is largely due to the commercial sector and is solely chicken based. Less-favored rural areas and dis-advantaged families, which account for 70% of Indian population are not benefited by this boom. Targeting small-scale, family-based poultry systems as an effective entry point for poverty alleviation programme is gaining widespread acceptance. Importance of the traditional system of poultry production is being rediscovered by researchers and development scientists.

Alternate poultry species have their regional/ seasonal importance. Further these alternate poultry species make the poultry production more diversified hence provide much diverse range of egg/meat products. Self reliant and hardy indigenous guinea fowl has adequate potential for becoming a crucial and integral part of the rural poultry production part. Guinea fowl may be a tailor made-germplasm for the rural poultry production system for the reasons being resistant to common chicken diseases, hardy and well adapted even under the adverse environmental conditions, excellent foraging ability and herd instinct and its integration with agriculture and horticulture. This species is studied at genetical and molecular level to a lesser extent. This book provides the information on these aspects of guinea fowl.

This book focuses on different aspects of the genetics of guinea fowl such as quantitative and qualitative genetics, cytogenetics, immuno-genetics and molecular genetics. It is hoped that this book on genetics and breeding of the guinea fowl will prove very useful to the researchers and teachers.

Deepak Sharma
Harpreet Singh

About the Editors

Dr Deepak Sharma, Ph.D. has worked for more than 25 years in poultry genetics and breeding. For last 12 years, he was engaged in guinea fowl breeding and also in Immuno-genetics as well as on Molecular Genetics. Presently he is Head, Animal Genetics Division, Indian Veterinary Research Institute, Izatnagar (UP). He has published more than 120 research articles. He may be contacted at ds7758@yahoo.co.in

Dr Harpreet Singh is retired Principal Scientist from Central Avian Research Institute, Izatnagar, Uttar Pradesh and at present is a consultant. He has worked on Blood polymorphism, Biochemical polymorphism in large animals as well as in poultry. He initiated research programmes on guinea fowl improvement at CARI and worked more than 13 years on guinea fowl.

Introduction

Poultry industry in India has a strong standing globally, being third highest egg producer with more than 54000 million eggs and fifth highest broiler producer with 2.5 million tones of broiler meat. Largely, Indian poultry industry is chicken dominated and rearing of high yielding varieties under intensive rearing system is the back bone of its present face. Presently, broiler industry is pocing at a growth rate of 10 %, while egg production has a growth rate of ~6 %. With these growth rates, egg production is expected to be more than 100 billion by 2020 and broiler production will be 8.6 million tones. However, these estimates may not be able to meet out the ever increasing demand of egg and meat.

Present growth in human population in India is estimated to be 1.404 % per year, against the average growth rate of 1.184 % in total Asian population and 0.906 % in world population. At this rate, the human population is expected to be 1173.8 million in India, 4149 million in Asia and 6830 million in World at the end of 2020. Existing growth rate in egg and poultry meat production will make the availability of 76 eggs per person per year in 2020. Similarly the availability of poultry peat per person per year will be 5.62 Kg by 2020.

Gap in requirement and supply

At the present level of production and per capita availability of eggs and poultry meat, India is far behind even fulfilling the recommendations of NIN which are 180 eggs per person per year and 11 kg meat per person per year. Existing per capita availability of eggs and poultry meat is about 2.0 kg poultry meat and < 40 eggs per person per year. To meet out the NIN requirement, the existing levels of egg production and poultry meat production should be 234000 million eggs and 12 millions tones of poultry meat, which are about 5-6 times more than the current production levels. These levels are difficult to achieve, but this gap can be narrowed by increasing the poultry production by adopting multifarious approaches. First need is to identify the short falls and lacuna and then to adopt the corrective measures.

Constraints

There are several well identified constraints which affect the growth of poultry adversely. These constraints are :

- Chicken dominated poultry production
- Pocketed poultry development
- High prices of conventional feed ingredients
- Seasonal fluctuations in consumption and prices of egg and meat
- Vegetarian feed habits especially in northern and western regions of country
- Lack of proper marketing channels
- Wet marketing of poultry meat

Strategy for increase in egg and poultry meat production

The wide gap exists between the current availability of egg and poultry meat and the recommended requirements can be bridged in principle by increasing the production and also be decreasing the losses in production. Increase in production can be achieved by increasing the number of birds as well as by improving the productivity of the birds. Therefore, a three tier can be adopted.

- Expansion of high input intensive chicken production system
- Reorienting and strengthening the Rural poultry production system
- Developing diversified poultry production system

Guinea Fowl for diversified poultry production

Guinea Fowl, one of the economically important avian species, is scientifically known as *Numida meleagris*. These guinea fowl are commonly known as helmeted guinea fowl. Originating from Africa, Guinea fowl were introduced into the Indian sub-continent during the slavery era of mediaeval centuries.

Preliminary survey of guinea fowl showed its distinct popularity with marginal farmers and other vulnerable groups as small-scale poultry enterprise. The indigenous germplasm seems well adapted to the diversified agro-climatic conditions prevailing in semi-arid regions. Guinea fowl population rank third after chickens and ducks. Guinea fowl may be a tailor-made germplasm for the rural poultry production system for the following reasons.

- The guinea fowl is resistant to common chicken diseases, hence do not require any health measures for their livability.
- It is hardy and well adapted even under the adverse environmental conditions.
- Guinea fowls have foraging ability and herd instinct, hence can easily be managed during foraging.
- Guinea fowl stock can be very well regenerated at the farmers level, hence the availability of replacement stock do not present a serious problem.
- Guinea fowl rearing can be used to control weeds, pests and ticks and other insects.

Guinea fowl is less explored poultry species; however information on different aspects of genetics is important for proper utilization of the genetic worth of guinea fowl. Hence in present book, we have tried to present information of genetics and breeding of guinea fowl. While the first two chapters are on Origin and domestication of guinea fowl and description of other species/ subspecies/ varieties of guinea fowl, other chapters are on Cytogenetics, Qualitative Genetics, Quantitative Genetics, Immunogenetics and Molecular Genetics.

❑❑❑

Chapter **1**

Origin and Domestication

Domestication and Early History

Domestication history of eco-friendly, traditional poultry farming genetic resource has high academic relevance. Guinea fowl, an integral part of African pastoral nomadics were possibly domesticated for aesthetic appeal and for religious rites as sacrifice to the deities as a sacred bird. The domestication history of guinea fowl within the African continent is not known very clearly, but its association with human beings has a curious career. It is generally agreed that two different guinea fowl species were independently domesticated at two different places but which one African people initiated domestication is not known clearly. These two regions were southern Sudan and West Africa. Depiction of guinea fowl in an Egyptian mural of about 2400 BC and archaeological remains found at Farnak (about 1900 B.C.) and Thebes (1570-1300 B.C.) indicate its importance.

By 400 B.C. guinea fowl were common barnyard poultry species in Greece and Greek islands. The 'Historia Naturallis' of Gaius Plinus Secundus (23 to 79 A.D.) also known as "Pliny the elder" presents the first reference of guinea fowl in Greece and it was referred as "Numida chicken". In Greek mythology, the grey breasted guinea fowl was referred as 'melanargis' meaning black and white, which was subsequently distorted and became meleagris'. The advent of guinea fowl to Greece is usually attributed to Carthaginian neighbors who had frequent contact with West-African neighbors. Wood-Gush (1985) suggests that the Moroccan sub-species Numida meleagris sabi was kept as a scared bird on an Augean island in the fourth century B.C. It was offered as sacrifice to the Athena. Later, Romans referred this bird as the Numidean fowl. They also had the birds of East-African sub-species named Meleagris and which they preferred. Both terms were subsequently utilized by Linnaeus in formal naming of the genus and species. Guinea fowl were highly regarded poultry food item throughout the Roman Empire (Zeuner 1963). It is difficult to guess why its popularity declined with the fall of Roman Empire. Only few references of the ensuing period texts indicate that the bird was domesticated by the ancients (Mongin and Plouzeau1983).

It is generally agreed that guinea fowl were reintroduced and disseminated from the west – Coastal African Gambian region by Portuguese traders during the later-half of fifteenth century tinto Europe, West Indies, Central America, India and Malaysia. In a way, all present day domestic guinea fowl are the descendents of these reintroductions (Somes 1996). Possibly, its present English name guinea (pronounced as "GINHEE") has been derived from a "Berber" would mean the "Land of Blacks". West African subspecies, Numida meleagris galeata, dispersed by the Portugese in most of the part of world is believed to be the ancestor of nearly all modern guinea fowl found in Europe, America and Asia. But the guinea fowl in Malagasy and those introduced from there to other localities may be domesticated Numida meleagris mitrata. Similarly, domestic guinea fowl found in eastern Africa are likely to be domesticates of meleagris and somaliensis subspecies, and those of the Mediterranean area may still bear traces of both East and West African subspecies.

Present Scenario of Guinea Fowl Production

Guinea fowl has a global distribution. The domesticated guinea fowl population found in Africa and some Asian countries including India are still close to their ancestor in behaviour as well as production potential. After the domestication, they have not received much attention either in term of their development as high yielding germplasm for meat production or egg production. Hence in these countries, these birds are reared under free range system or under semi-intensive system in the areas where some attention was paid by the Extension organizations or NGOs. But the population in Europe and Russia, were improved for meat and/or egg production and they are being reared under large commercial setups. In Europe, France and Italy are the main countries rearing the millions of guinea fowl under intensive system. Soviet Union and Hungary also has large scale guinea fowl production.

National Scenario of Guinea Fowl

In India, guinea fowl population ranks third after chickens and ducks. Guinea fowl is referred by different regional names in this subcontinent, e.g. 'Chittra' in the western regions, 'Titari' in northern plains; and 'Chinha Murgi' (Cheena Murgi) in the southern peninsular and eastern parts. Earliest attempts to raise guinea fowl under intensive conditions were made at the Christian Missionary Poultry Farm, Etah (UP); Allahabad Agriculture Institute, Naini (UP); Government Poultry Farm, Gurdaspur (Punjab) and subsequently at the Millitary Poultry Farms also.

A preliminary survey of guinea fowl production in northern India and the perusal of earlier published literature established its distinct popularity with marginal farmers and other vulnerable groups as small scale poultry enterprise and an opportunity to diversify (Singh and Panda 1984). Raised as free-range poultry with minimal inputs, the indigenous germplasm seems well adapted to diversified agro-climatic conditions prevailing in arid and semi-arid regions. The traditional popularity of guinea fowl is generally attributed to its hardiness, disease resistance and ability to survive and thrive under low management and feeding conditions.

Although organised enterprise is practically nonexistent but flocks of 150 to 200 or more heads on droving is a common site in guinea fowl producing pockets (Fig 1.1). Definite population figures are not available; perhaps a few million birds are raised every year. Its meat and eggs have ready acceptability in all the production pockets.

The prevailing socio-economic conditions of Indian small farmers strongly underline - the need for development of the low-input grain saving aviculture systems.

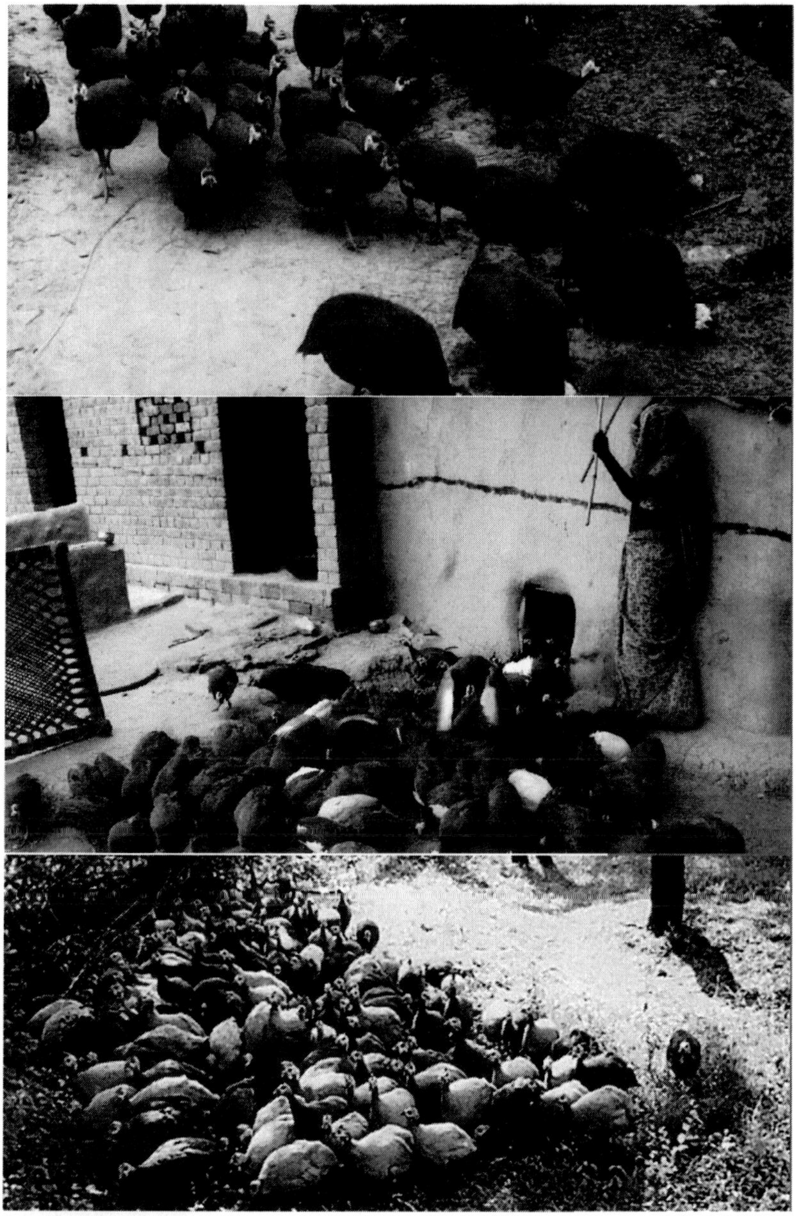

Fig. 1.1 :

❐❐❐

Chapter **2**

Species and Varieties

Classification

The guinea fowl is a bird under the order - Galliformes, class - Aves, Phylum - Chordata and Kingdom - Animalia. Guinea fowls make a separate family - Numididae, under the order Galliformes, but the American Ornithologists' Union placed the guinea fowl, as a sub-species, Numidinae under the family Phasianidae. However, the former classification is more widely accepted and used. There are four genera of the family Numididae i.e. Agelastes, Guttera, Numida and Acryllium. Under each genus, there are one or more species.

Genus	Species	Common name
Agelastes	*Agelastes meleagrides*	White-breasted Guinea fowl
	Ageiastes niger	Black Guinea fowl
Guttera	*Guttera plumifera*	Plumed Guinea fowl
	Guttera pucherani	Crested Guinea fowl
Acryllium	*Acryllium vulturinum*	Vulturine Guinea fowl
Numida	*Numida meleagris*	Helmeted Guinea fowl

Agelastes genus

Guinea fowl under this genus have no crest or helmet. These are smallest among all the Guinea fowls. The head and neck are bare and naked skin has wrinkles and is rose red in clour. Plumage is black. These Guinea fowl are native to damp forests of Ghana and Liberis. There are two species in this genus. Agelastes meleagride is small sized bird having black plumage. Mantle and breast are white, hence also known as White breasted guinea fowl. It is found in Ghana and Liberia. Agelastes nige is another species of guinea fowl under this genus and is found in tropical rain forests of Ghana and lower Guinea. It has a small body and black plumage, hence also known as Black guinea fowl.

Guttera genus

Guinea fowl under Guttera genus are characterized by the presence of thick bunch of inky black feathers and brilliantly coloured featherless skin of head and neck. There are two species i.e. Guttera plumifera (Plumed Guinea fowl) and Guttera pucherani (Crested Guinea fowl). While Guttera plunifera hibitates in Cameroon or Gabon, Guttera pucherani is found in Kenya, Sierra Leoone, Angola or Natal.

Acryllium genus

These guinea fowl are the largest among all other guinea fowls. It is found in southern Ethiopia, Somalia and East Africa. It has a bare and blue head and white spotted black plumage. Neck, legs and tail are longer than other Guinea fowl. It gives an "vulture like" resemblance due to its long neck and hooked beak. The slim neck projects from a cape of long, glossy, blue and white hackles. The breast is cobalt blue, and the rest of the body plumage is black, finely spangled with white. There is one species in this genus i.e. Acryllium vulturinum, also known as vulturine Guinea fowl.

Numida genus

Guinea fowl under genus Numida are characterized by the presence of a bony structure on the head, known as helmet, hence these are also known as helmeted guinea fowl.

It is found in Africa, mainly south of the Sahara, and has been widely introduced into the West Indies and southern France. It is a large bird with a round body and small head. The body plumage is gray-black spangled with white spots. Round the mantle, a reddish violet band is present. Head is feather less. The wings are short and rounded, and the tail is also short. There is only one species in this genus i.e. Numida meleagris, also known as grey breasted or helmeted guinea fowl.

Helmeted Guinea fowl *(Numida meleagris)*

Several sub species have been reported under this family, however Crowe (1985) has classified them into nine well marked subspecies (Table 2.1).

Table 2.1 : Sub species of helmeted guinea fowl

West African	*Numida meleagris galeata* *Numida meleagris sabyi*
East African	*Numida meleagris meleagris* *Numida meleagris somaliensis*
Central-South African	*Numida meleagris reichenowi* *Numida meleagris mitrata* *Numida meleagris marungensis* *Numida meleagris papillosa* *Numida meleagris coronata*

Among these seven subspecies, Numida meleagris galeata is the principal ancestor of the domestic guinea fowl. It is found throughout West Africa. There is much variation in the size and other characteristics within the subspecies. It is small to medium sized, have naked cere and rounded red wattles. Another subspecies, Numida meleagris sabyi found as an isolated northern population in Morocco resembles closely with the Numida meleagris galeata. Among the East African subspecies, Numida meleagris meleagris, also known as tufted guinea fowl have quite large body and has black plumage thickly spotted with white dots. It has long bristles on the cere and rounded blue wattles. This subspecies is reared in southern Sudan. Another subspecies of East Africa is Numida meleagris somaliensis and it also has medium-sized body, long bristles on the cere and rounded blue wattles. Central-South African group are relatively large birds, have a naked cere (except for Numida meleagris papillosa which has warts around the rim) and triangular-shaped blue wattles with red tips. Numida meleagris mitrata also known as Mitred guinea fowl is the most popular game bird. It has a blue green head and red wattle. It is found in Kenya and Tanzania. Indigenous population found in Yemen is similar to East African subspecies, for which some authors have classified it as separate species i.e. Numida ptilorhyncha or blue wattled guinea fowl.

Confirmation and Terminology

Common guinea fowl are medium sized, compact bodied gallinaceous birds. As yet, no standards of perfection have been fixed for different varieties. The points considered important are good size and uniformity in plumage colour.

Head: Large, obvate and sturdy head is adorned with a characteristic hard bony bump the 'helmet'. The head has only few feathers or non at all. Eyes are small, deeply set but bright and alert. Skin under eyes and the ear lobes has white patches. Beak is short and stout, attached somewhat low on the head, wattles are red with whitish patch at one on each side of the beak.

Neck: Fairly long and tapering neck is carried mainly upwards and forwards. It is bare near the head but the lower part has great deal of white skin about it and a thin mane of bristles behind.

Beak: It is short, stout, rounded and tapers rapidly towards the tip.

Tail: Fairly short, compact and droopy tail has fourteen feathers, usually heavily over laid with upper tail coverts.

Wings: Strong rounded and well developed wings also have strong muscles. Younger birds possess good ability to fly with agility and roost high off the ground.

Body: Broad-shouldered and well rounded body is rather proportioned to semicircular dimensions of the back and underlines. The low carriage of sternum anddownwords profile of the back provides the guinea fowl an almost circular appearance.,

Legs: Typical for all game birds, the guinea legs are long and well set apart with hocks showing below the thigh covers. Strong legs of sufficient length make these birds very suitable for scavenging and grazing.

Plumage: In full plumage these are fluffy and present deceptively larger looks than the actual size. Many feather colour variations like; violet, liliac, buff (chamois), white etc all with or without spotting might be seen. But dark grey coloured plumage, evenly speckled with light dotts (pearl) is distinctive and very common. Young keets in down also present a distinctive pattern of light and dark markings. In dark plumaged varieties, the skin and skin formation namely leg scales and beak are also dark.

Guinea fowl Varieties

Description of breeds and varieties are generally the description of populations. The term 'variety' refers to a groups of birds identical in all characteristics except plumage colour, weight, colour of shanks or some other minor details. Unlike chicken, not many varieties are known for guinea fowl. The existing varieties are classified according to plumage colour. The three principal well known varieties are the Pearl, White and Lavender (Fig 2.1). Other plumage mutations were also described in literature including White-Breasted, Buff, Royal-purple and the Coral-blue etc.

Pearl: Most common and popular, the pearl variety appears to have developed originally from the wild African type. Plumage is uniformly dark grey in colour, regularly sprinkle with dots which give it the characteristic pearled appearance. These uniformly distributed spots are usually, but not invariably large and round. In some birds these spots may be absent and this grey non-spotted variety is called violet. Presence of white flight feathers is a common defect. The keets of this variety resemble young quails. Their first feathers are brown while under part of the body might be lighter than the rest. The beak and legs are reddish in colour. These brown feathers gradually disappear by about two months of age and finally get completely replaced by the typical 'pearled' feathers.

Lavender: The birds of this variety are light gray or lavender in colour and always uniformly dotted with white. The presence of white feathers is not favoured in pure specimen. This variety is more popular in Italy. The lavender and white guinea are considered more adaptable to colder regions. Perhaps these are relatively less susceptible to winter snow bites.

White: This variety is characterized by presence of completely white plumage. It has a lighter skin than Pearl variety. In some countries, white variety is preferred over others. In Russia, white variety has been improved for meat.

White breasted variety: This variety is characterized by pearl plumage with white breast feathers. This plumage pattern is produced by crossing the white and pearl or lavender varieties, hence these variety do not breed true. This variety is also known as splashed.

Other varieties: Buff, Coral-blue, Dundottes, Isabellia, Liliac, Royal purple are other plumage patterns.

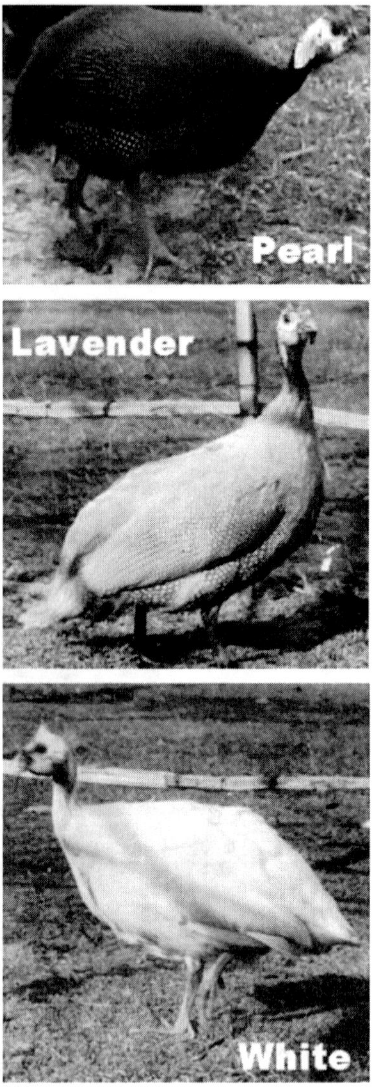

Fig. 2.1

Chapter **3**

Cytogenetics

Chromosomes

Chromosome may be defined as an organized structure of DNA and protein that is present in nucleus of the cell. The chromosome word comes from the two Greek words i.e. *Chroma*, means colour and *soma*, means body. This name has been given due to its property of being heavily stained with certain dyes. In a normal cell, the chromosomes of eukaryotes exist as uncondensed DNA in a quasi-ordered structure inside the nucleus, wrapping around the histones. The double stranded DNA (200 bp) wrapped around an octomer of histones (comprising of 2 molecules each of H2A, H2B,

H3 and H4) and one molecule of H1 which acts as anchor, forms one nucleosome. This structure is 10 nm in diameter and is referred as primary structure of chromosome. The chromatin fiber is a flexibly joined chain of nucleosomes which can be folded into a 20-30 nm fiber probably by forming a solenoidal structure having six nucleosomes per turn and is referred as secondary structure of chromosome. The chromatin fiber then makes a loop like structures radiating in all the direction from a central protein core. A group of six loops, radiating from one central protein core make one hexameric rosette and is about 200-300 nm in diameter. This loop like organization of chromatin makes tertiary structure of chromosome. The quarternary structure is formed by further coiling of the rosette and one coil includes 30 rosette. The number of coils in one chromosome is dependent upon the amount of DNA present in that chromosome (Fig 3.1).

Two types of chromatin is distinguishable in resting cell i.e. euchromatin and heterochromatin. Euchromatin consists of DNA that is active, e.g., expressed as protein. Heterochromatin consists of mostly inactive DNA. It seems to serve structural purposes during the chromosomal stages.

Heterochromatin can be further distinguished into two types i.e. *Constitutive heterochromatin*, which is never expressed. It is located around the centromere and usually contains repetitive sequences, and *Facultative heterochromatin*, which is sometimes expressed.

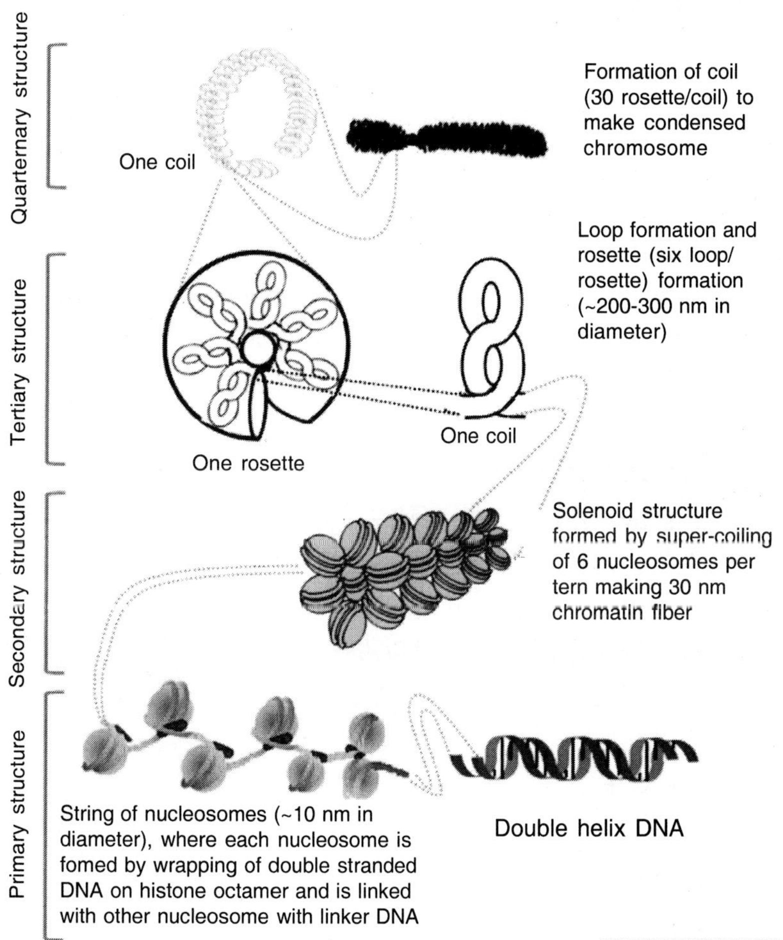

Fig. 3.1 : Different levels of chromosome structure

During the early phase of cell division, the chromosome starts organizing itself into highly condensed shape. The typical shape of the chromosome has a constriction point called the centromere, which divides the chromosome into two arms. The short arm of the chromosome is known as p arm and the long arm of the chromosome is known as q arm. Chromosomes are the essential unit for cellular division and must be replicated, divided, and passed successfully to their daughter cells so as to ensure the inheritance of the genetic information from parents to offspring as well as for growth. Hence to understand the certain phenomenon of genetics in a better way, the process of cell division should be clearly known.

Cell and Cell division

Cells are the basic biological units. Theoretically an adult fowl can be resolved into about eight to ten billion (8-10^{14}) somatic and germ line cells. Even though highly differentiated to perform specific functions, all cells share common features viz. the outer envelope, cytoplasm with its organelles, and a nucleus having fixed number of homologous chromosome pairs: one from each of the two parents. All cells originate from pre-existing living cells. The two processes of cell reproduction i.e. Mitosis (for somatic cells) and Meiosis (for germ cells) are fundamental basis of animal reproduction. In higher class of organisms including poultry, the generation of the progeny occurs through fusion of sex cells (sperm from male and ova from female). Therefore to maintain the same number of chromosomes in progenies, the number of chromosomes in sex cells is to be reduced to half of the parental chromosome number. This reduction of chromosome number takes place through meiotic cell division, while mitotic cell division provide the basis of growth or multiplication through increase in cell number without reducing chromosomes number from parental cell to new cells. During any cell division, each individual cell passes through a well-defined cell cycle i.e. Interphase or rest-phase and active cell division phase (M). Interphase is consists of G_0, G_1, S and G_2 stages. The G_0 and G_1 phases are the pre DNA-synthesis phase, however the latter phase marks preparatory phase of chromosomes to divide. During the synthetic phase (S), deoxyribose nucleic acid (DNA) is replicated and whole chromosome compliment (2n) is duplicated (4n), which is followed by the post-synthetic gap phase (G_2). Cell will remain in G_0 until conditions become conductive for initiation of division. Duration of these phases of Interphase vary not only in different species, but also vary in different tissues from same organism (Fig 3.2).

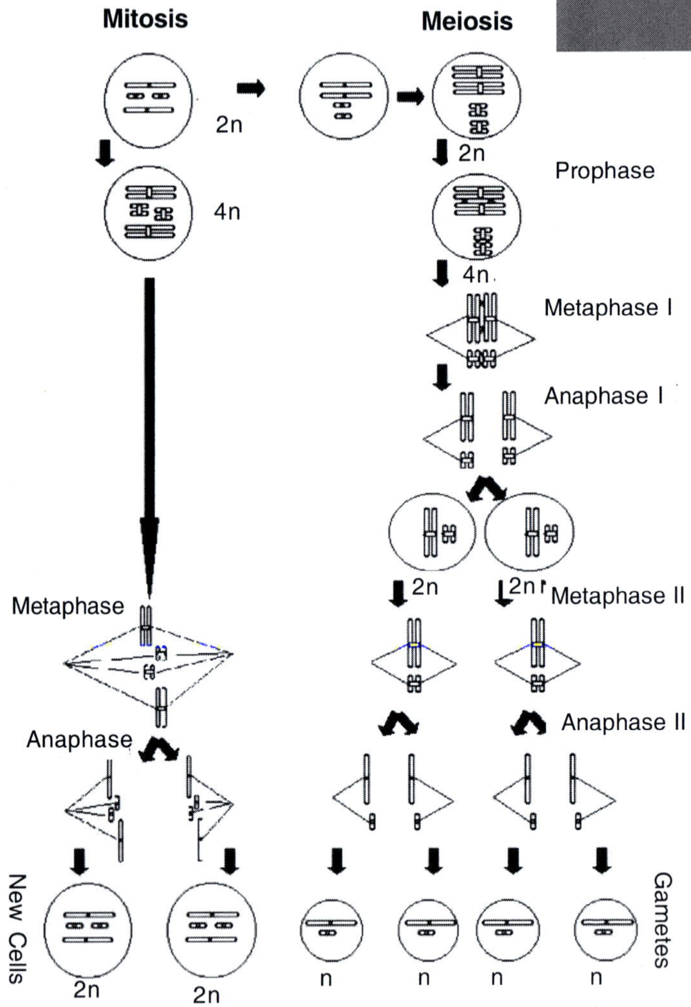

Fig. 3.2 : Different stages of cell division

Mitosis

Mitosis is observed where number of somatic cells are increasing during growth or when dead cells are being replaced. The timing and initiation of mitosis depends on the G2 phase that takes place after the complete duplication of chromosomes. Mitosis is subdivided into four cytological phases viz. the prophase, metaphase, anaphase and telophase. In prophase, chromosomes condense and become visible as pairs of chromatids, while spindle formation and subsequent alignment of chromosomes at the equator characterize the metaphase. Anaphase is identified by the separation of two chromatids of each chromosome, followed by their migration to the two poles. Finally, the telophase marks the completion of cell division and formation of two diploid daughter cells identical with the original cell.

Meiosis

Meiosis is very complex but highly ordered division process during which diploid chromosome (2n) number is reduced to haploid (n) number. The cell chromosome complement first divide and segregate into homologous (identical) pairs. These cells with 4n chromosomes subsequently divide twice resulting into formation of four cells which contain half the original number of chromosomes i.e. the haploid set. This reduction of chromosome number during the formation of gametes is essential for maintenance of the species-specific constant chromosome number from generation to generation. Meiosis allows for genetic variation and ensures thorough reshuffling of homologous chromosomes from each parent before one of each pair is randomly assigned to each new cell. Thus the theoretically possible number of combination for a species with haploid set (n) of 39 chromosomes may be as high as 239. The breaking of parental linkage groups through chiasama formations further ensure that haploid cells resulting from meiosis will have variable combinations of genes. Meiosis also serves as a screening process through selection of genetically unfit cell lines where deficiencies and deletions cause genomic imbalance in large animals.

Morphology of Chromosome

Since the chromosome are visible as well as distinguishable at the time of cell division only, most of the knowledge about the chromosomes has come from study of the metaphase chromosomes. The condensed chromosome has two arms i.e. short arm and long arm and a central region, where these arms are attached. This is also the form in which chromosome is generally diagrammatically shown. After replication, the chromosomes appears as a X shape structure, having four microtubules joined in center. The replicated chromatids are called sister chromatids. Typically a chromosome (Fig 3.3) may have all or some of the following structures.

Chromatids: Chromatids are the tubular structure, originating after condensation of chromatin into higher degree of organization.

Centromere: It is primary constriction point, which divides the chromosome into two sections, or "arms." The short arm of the chromosome is labeled the "p arm." The long arm of the chromosome is labeled the "q arm". The centeromere are found to have certain specific DNA sequences. Some special proteins bind to them and forms a disc like structure at centromere, known as kinetochore.

Teleomere: These are called the end-cap of chromosome and present on the extreme end of chromatid. It is composed of DNA and protein.

Secondary Constriction: Chromosome may have one or more constrictions apart from primary constriction (at centromere). It may be long or short. Certain secondary constriction possess genes coding for 5.8S, 18S and 28S ribosomal rRNA.

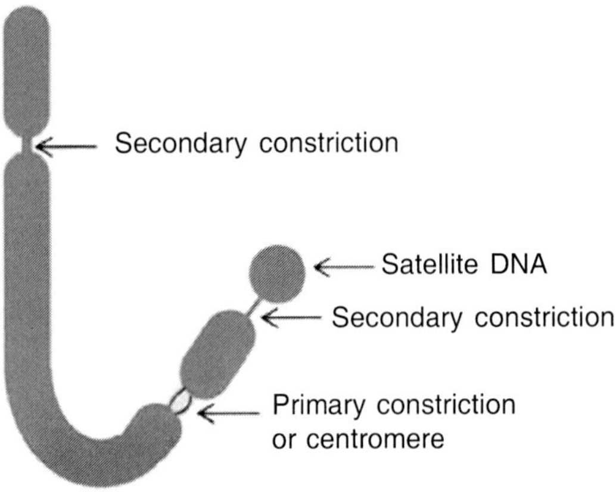

Fig. 3.3 : Structure of a typical chromosome

Satellite: It is the round elongated body, may be of the same diameter as that of chromosome formed due to secondary constriction.

Nucleolar organisers: It is the chromosomal region possessing genes coding for 5.8S, 18S and 28S ribosomal rRNA and it induces the nucleoli formation. Generally this region is found in satellited chromosomes as in human, but this association is not universal.

The general morphology of a chromosome depends upon the dimensions of the chromosomes, position of the centromere and the presence of other structures like secondary constriction and satellites. The chromosomes may be classified on the basis of the position of centromere and may be metacentric, submetacentric, acrocentric or telocentric (Fig 3.4).

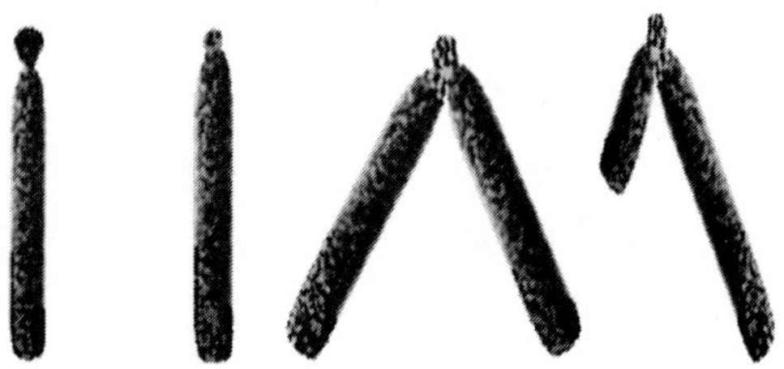

Fig. 3.4 : Different types of chromosomes based on position of centeromere

The Telocentric chromosomes are rod shaped, having centromere at the terminal end, thus it has only one arm. Acrocentric chromosome also possesses the rod shape, but have centromere closer to one end of chromosome, thus one arm is very short as compared to other one. In Metacentric chromosomes, centromere is located in centre, resulting in equal sized arms. These chromosomes have 'V'-shape. The submetacentric chromosomes are 'L' or 'J' shaped, having centromere somewhat away from the centre, thus both the chromatids are of not equal size.

The 'n' number of chromosome refers to the total chromosomes present in cell. Since at the time of sexual cell division (meiosis), the identical chromosomes make pairs and are called homologous chromosomes. These homologous chromosomes are not only identical in size, but also carry the same alleles or different alleles of the same genes. The number of pairs of chromosome present in cell is called as '2n' number of chromosomes. Sometimes 'n' and 2n numbers are also called as haploid and diploid number.

Autosome and Sex chromosome

In a diploid cell, all the chromosomes, except sex chromosomes appeared in pair and both the chromosome of a pair are called homologous chromosomes. These chromosomes are known as autosomes and in both the sexes i.e. male and female, they are same or homomorphic. However, sex chromosomes are not same in both the sexes and may be homomorphic in one sex and heteromorphic in other sex. In mammalians, for sex chromosomes, XX or XY system is used. The females are XX i.e. homomorphic, while males are XY i.e. heteromorphic (Fig 3.5).

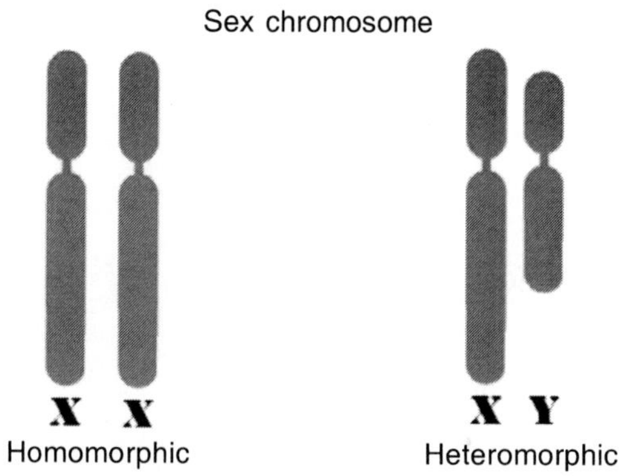

Fig. 3.5 : Diagrammatic representation of mammalian sex chromosomes

Banding of chromosomes

Staining of the chromosomes with different stains produces the different type of banding patterns. These patterns are important for identification of the chromosomes, mapping the different regions including genes on the chromosome etc. Normally staining is dome at metaphase stage of cell division.

G banding: Staining of the chromosome (at metaphase stage) with the giemsa stain after treating it with trypsin (to partly digest the chromosome) generate a series of alternating light and dark bands called G bands (Fig 3.6).

Fig. 3.6 : Diagrammatic representation of G banding pattern

The dark band reveals the regions tend to be heterochromatic, late-replicating and highly AT rich, while the light regions tend to be euchromatic, early-replicating and GC rich. The G bands are numbered and provide the positions of different genes mapped on the chromosome.

C banding: C banding is produced through treatment of metaphase chromosome with hydrochloric acid followed by sodium/barium hydrochloride, incubation in a warm salt water and staining with Giemsa. This banding is used to define the constitutive hetrochromatin, hence it stain centromere.

R banding: Heating of chromosomes in a phosphate buffer and subsequent staining with Giemsa stain produces the banding pattern that is the reverse of that produced in G-banding i.e. dark regions are euchromatic (guanine-cytosine rich regions) and the bright regions are heterochromatic (thymine-adenine rich regions).

Q banding: It is a fluorescent pattern produced by quinacrine staining. The pattern of bands is very similar to G-banding.

T-banding: T-banding is used to stain the telomeric regions of chromosomes and is produced by controlled thermal denaturation followed by staining with either Giemsa or acridine orange. The T bands apparently represent a subset of the R bands because they are smaller that the corresponding R bands and are more strictly telomeric.

RE banding: It is produced by restriction enzumes and is similar to that of G and C banding.

Silver staining: It is used to stains the nucleolar organization region-associated protein. This yields a dark region where the silver is deposited, denoting the activity of rRNA genes within the NOR.

Karyotype

The whole collection of the chromosomes in a nucleus is referred as karyotype or chromosome complement. The karyotype is the characteristic of an individual, species, genus or may be order. The karyotype may be symmetrical or asymmetrical. In animal kingdom, asymmetrical karyotypes are almost universal. The diagrammatic representation of the karyotype showing all the morphological features of the chromosomes is known as idiogram. In idiogram only one chromosome of an autosomal chromosome pairs is showed, while for sex chromosome pair, both the chromosomes are showed (Fig 3.7). All chromosomes of a complement are numbered in descending order of size as per the standard methods developed for numbering.

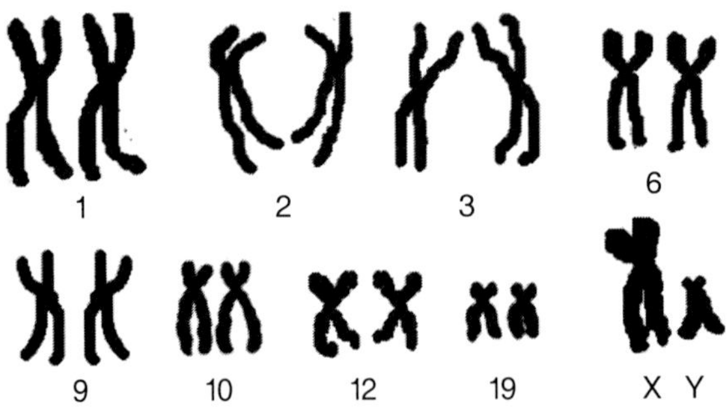

Fig. 3.7 : Diagrammatic representation of karyotype

Avian chromosome complement

In Aves, the chromosomes are conventionally divided into two subsets: the macro-chromosomes (MACS) which are large in size and few in numbers and large number of small sized individually indistinguishable the micro-chromosomes (MICS). It is an arbitrary grouping, and opinions differ regarding the definition of these two subsets since any sharp border line demarcating these two groups is rarely observed among the gallinaceous species. One more characteristic of the avian species is the heterogametic female (ZW) and homogametic male (ZZ), in contrast to heterogametic male (XY) and homogametic female (XX). The chromosome number (n and 2n), number of macro and microchromosomes and sex chromosome in different domesticated poultry species are as follows

Table 3.1 : Number of chromosomes in different poultry species

Species	Chromosome Numbers		MACS (2n)	MICS (2n)
	n	2n		
Guinea fowl (numida meleagidris)	78	39	8	31
Chicken (Gallus domesticus)	78	39	8	31
Japanes quail (Coturnix coturnix))	78	39	6	33
Turkey (Meleagris gallipavo)	80	40	6	34
Domestic duck (Anna latyrhynchos)	78	39	6	33
Goose (Anesr anser)	80	40	6	34

Guinea fowl chromosome complement

Macro-chromosomes (MACS): The model chromosome number for guinea fowl is 78. Though there is no distinct bi-modality between macro and micro-chromosomes. The first five pair of chromosomes are considered as macro-chromosomes (MACS), 6th to 8th pairs as large micro-chromosomes (Large MICS) remaining pairs as unidentifiable microchromosomes (MICS). Their morphometric attributes are summarized in Table 3.2. Among the macro-chromosomes, the size ratio of largest to smallest macro-chromosomes is 4.7:1.0. According to size and arm-ratio these chromosomes are divisible into three groups : the first group included of 1st, 2nd and 4th pair of sub-metacentric chromosomes, the former two pairs obviously are the largest; the second group included 3rd and 7th pairs of acrocentric chromosomes while the metacentric 6th pair formed the third group. Observations differ only with respect to morphology of the 3rd chromosome which was also described acrocentric, perhaps it needs further confirmation. The first three chromosome pairs constitute about 54.0% of the genome.

Guinea fowl male is homogametic (ZZ) sex, and the Z chromosome is conspicuous sub-metacentric and fifth largest in order. Female is heterogametic (ZW) sex and the W chromosome is acrocentric, small and not readily distinguishable from other micro-chromosomes. It is identified due to its small size and the positive C-band, the areas of constitutive (permanently inner) hetrochromatin. The Z chromosome pair of male chromosome complement constitutes about 10.6 percent of the genome.

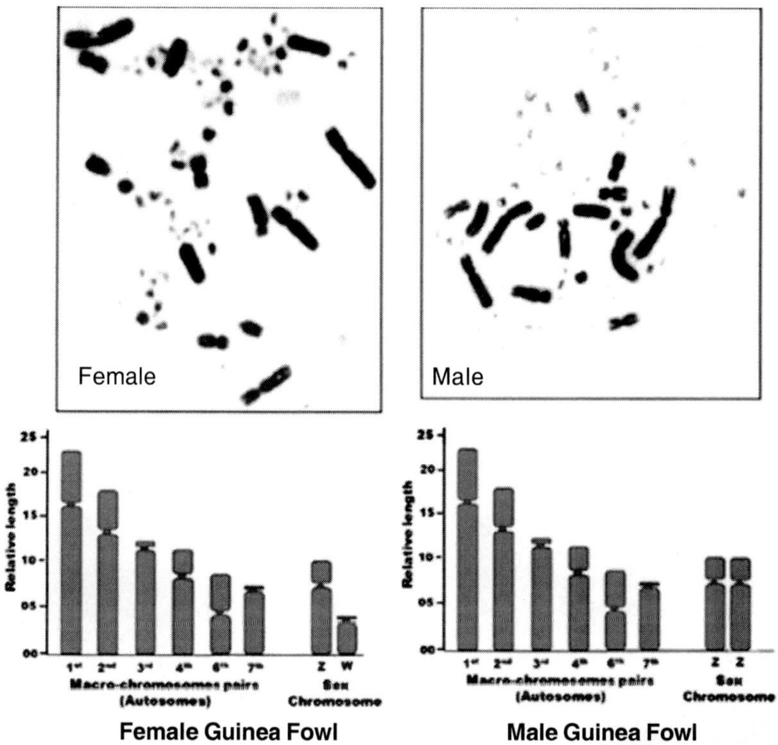

Fig. 3.8 : Metaphase chromosome spread in male and female guinea fowl and diagrammatic representation of the sizes of macro-chromosomes including sex chromosomes.

Micro-chromosomes (MICS): Although 58 to 64 micro-chromosomes (MICS) have been reported in literature, but 64 is considered as standard number. Except for small size, all the micro-chromosomes are true chromosomes. Their large array form a continuous gradation, the smallest one could hardly be distinguished from the largest micro bivalent and most of MICS show terminal centromeres. These karyotype

Table 3.2 : Relative length (RL) and CI estimates for different macro-chromosomes in guinea fowl and chicken.

MACS	Guinea Fowl		Domestic Fowl	
	RL	CI	RL	CI
1st	23.0 ± 0.6 (SM)	37.7 ± 1.7	25.2 ± 0.5 (SM)	40.6 ± 1.0
2nd	18.6 ± 0.1 (SM)	36.0 ± 1.6	19.21 ± 0.4 (SM)	35.9 ± 1.42
3rd	12.6 ± 0.5 (AC)	-	14.5 ± 0.3 (AC)	-
4th	12.3 ± 0.3 (SM)	32.3 ± 6.2	11.5 ± 0.3 (SM)	19.3 ± 1.5
5th	10.6 ± 0.5 (M)	43.7 ± 1.7	11.7 ± 0.3 (M)	19.3 ± 2.9
6th	8.8 ± 0.5 (M)	48.8 ± 2.4	07.7 ± 0.3 (AC)	-
7th	7.5 ± 0.4 (AC)	-	05.2 ± 0.3 (AC)	-
8th	4.1 ± 0.2 (AC)	-	04.9 ± 0.3 (AC)	28.5 ± 4.7

studies confirmed agreement to the modal ancestral chromosomal complement of six macro-chromosomes including the sex chromosomes identified for the gallinaceous birds i.e. 1,2,3,4/m, 5 and Z for macro-

chromosomes and also the large (70-76) number of micro-chromosomes (De Boyer 1984). The micro-chromosomes mainly consist of heterochromatin, genes located within heterochromatin are known to influence quantitative and physiological characters. But little is known about the effect of a loss or gain of heterochromatin material although existence of variability in micro-chromosome (MICS) number has been reported in several galliformes species.

Differential Banding Pattern

Observations regarding G-banding and C-banding patterns help in defining the chromosome features and identification of homologous chromosome. As per staining properties, areas of the chromosomes can be divided into euchromatin and heterochromatin. The euchromatin is diffuse and lightly straining in contrast to heterochromatin which is densely staining. The difference is due to compaction of chromatin; heterochromatin having more compact organization is believed not to be generally active in the process of transcription.

Banding pattern observations help in defining the internal organization of chromosome features and identification of homologous chromosomes. These provide a better understanding of chromosomal organization and rearrangement, addition or deletion of hetrochromatin material and accurate assessment of variation of closely related genetic groups. Limited studies of guinea fowl G-banding and C-banding pattern revealed no variant banding pattern. Structural variations of macro-chromosomes and chromosomal aberrations were also not observed (Stock and Bunch 1982, Ansari and Singh 1983, Goswami and Singh, 1990, 1996. Vijh et al. 1997).

Sister Chromatid Exchanges (SCE) and Nucleolar Organiser Regions (NOR)

Sister chromatid exchanges (SCE) and nucleolar orgnaiser regions (NOR) observations help identification of structural aberrations and chromosome lesions e.g. fragile sites, secondary constrictions gaps etc. The sister chromatid exchange frequency was found to be low about (1.71 per cell or 0.85 per cell per generation) since differential staining is observable only in case of macro chromosomes. The nucleolar organiser regions (NOR s) associated with nucleolus formation are specific sites on specific chromosomes, which represent multiple copies of r RNA genes associated with the ribosome functions. Terminal or interstitial NORs are diagnostic chromosome markers characteristic of species. In guinea fowl NORs were identified on a pair of micro-chromosomes by Vijh et al. (1997). Presence of NOR s in case of domestic fowl was observed on the 17th micro-chromosome which contains the major histocompatibility (MHC) locus. Although no detailed survey of the chromosomal complement of guinea fowl adults or embryos have been made but limited studies have not revealed alternations in the number of whole chromosomes from the 2n (heteropioidy) deficiency or excess of whole chromosomes (aneuploidy) duplications or deficiencies and aberrant chromosome forms (Piccini and Stella 1970, Denisove and Khrustalev 1974, Stock and Bunch 1982, Belterman and Boer 1984, Kozikova 1984, Goswami and Singh 1990, 1996, Vijh et al. 1997). High incidences of aberrant chromosomal forms have been reported in domestic fowl (Bitgood and Shoffner 1990).

Karyotypic differences vis-à-vis other galliforms

Karyotypic resemblances may or may not sufficiently reflect phylogenetic affinities but present comparison of guinea fowl macrochromosomes with that of chicken and quail (Ansari and Singh, 1983; Goswami and Singh, 1990; 1996) and also those reported for other gallinaceous species revealed an essential similarity between *Gallus, Numida* and *Coturnix* species. The identifiable chromosome pairs of guinea fowl revealed a size range comparable to that of chicken; the size ratios of largest to smallest chromosome of the two species e.g. Guinea fowl 5.7:1.0, Domestic fowl 5.1:1.0 was not different significantly. The observed morphological differences in macro-chromosomes could be explained on the basis of few peri-centric inversions and additions or deletions of some heterochromatic material. Guinea fowl differ from chicken by a centric fusion of two micro-chromosomes which formed a unique pair of additional metacentric autosome (*m/m-4*). Presence of an additional interstitial C-band on the long arm of chromosome *4/m* and relatively lower number of micro-chromosomes *vis-a-vis* that of chicken was characteristic. The observed chromosomal plan for guinea fowl and chicken agreed completely with that suggested earlier by Belterman and De Bore (1984) which could be described as 1, 2, 3, 4/m Co, 5, m/m4, Zinv and 1, 2, 3, 4/m, Zinv respectively.

□□□

Chapter **4**

Qualitative Genetics

Qualitative Genetics

Primary reason of all genetic studies is to identify inherited variations which may be discrete or continuous in nature. Qualitative genetics is the study of traits showing discontinuous variation i.e. they can be grouped as discrete classes. These traits are generally not influenced by environment and are governed by single or few genes under simple Mendelian inheritance. The examples of qualitative traits include simple phenotypic differences in plumage colour, skin colour, shank colour, feather development, other morphological features immunologically or biochemically identified differences etc.

A. Morphogeneic Polymorphism

The 'morph' refers to the discrete plumage type unrelated to age and occurrence in same inter-breeding population. Despite the extensive attention focused on plumage genes of domesticated avian species, not much is known about guinea fowl plumage morphogenetics.

Bright plumage colours and striking patterns are the most conspicuous morphorphological feature of avian species. Following the discovery of Mendelism, plumage phenotypes were among the first few characters that attracted the attention of poultry geneticists; since then a wide array of genes that influence structure, pattern, growth rate, ultimate size and also the major and minor plumage cover variations have been reported in domestic fowl and other poultry species. Discovery of these morphogenetic mutants have played an important role in poultry production development of breeds, strains and fancy varieties, the routine maintenance of breeds and synthesis of stocks for commercial exploitation.

In chicken large number of variants for feathering, comb, skin, skeleton and muscular systems are found and have been studied in depth. In brief, a large number of plumage pattern, primary as well as secondary are found. Some good examples of primary plumage pattern is black, dark brown or Columbian, while for secondary plumage patterns are barring, mottling or stippling. Similarly for feather distribution, the some well known variants are normal feathering, naked neck or ptilopody (feathers on feet), while for feather length, it is crest, muffs and long tail. Some good examples for feather structure variation are frizzling and silkiness, while the slow and early featherings are variants of growth of feathers. Different types of comb such as single, rose, pea combs and gene influencing them are very well known in chicken. For skin pigmentation, very well established variants are white and yellow skin, while some skin structure variants are ear tuft, enlarged ear lobe etc. There are certain more variations involving axial skeleton, which affect beak, head, neck and body (sparrow head/ crooked neck etc) as well as body size (dominant or recessive sex linked and autosomal dwarfism). In guinea fowl, the studies on these variants are very limited and some of the variants studied are discussed.

Plumage color gene

In some avian species, melanin and carotenoid pigments contribute to the plumage colour, but in domestic fowl, melanin solely determine the plumage colour. Melanin, a widespread natural pigment has major role in colour of skin, shank, shank, beak and eyes. There are two major types of melanin i.e. Eumelanin (found in black/ blue feathers, eye, skin and also tissues) and pheomelanin (found in red-brown, salmon and buff colored feathers. Carotenoids are not synthesized in the body of fowl. Main caretenoids found in the body of fowl is xanthophylls, which is yellow pigment and gives yellow colour to beak, skin, shank, iris of eye as well as to yolk of egg and body fat. The feed ingredients like yellow maize, alfalfa leaf meal etc are the main source of xanthophylls. In wild type, the genes are for normal production of both type of melanin i.e. eumelanin and phenomelanin, but the intra allelic as well as inter allelic interactions results in different plumage colour and pattern. The distribution pattern of eumelanin may be primary or secondary. While primary pattern shows the zonal or regional location of eumelanin resulting in few to many feather tracts, secondary pattern shows the distribution of eumelanin within individual feathers as barring, stippling etc. In chicken, polyallelic E locus is considered to determine the basic or zonal distribution of eumemanin. There are atlease eight alleles at E locus i.e. Extended Black (E), Birchen (ER), Dominant wheaten (eWh), Wild type (e+), Brown (eB), specked (es), Buttercap (ebc) and Recessive Wheaten (ey). While there are some genetic factors which intensify the eumelanization like eumelanin enhancer melanotic (Ml), other factors like some mutations acts as eumelanin inhibitor. Three well known eumelanin inhibitors are Columbian (C0), dark brown (Db) and mahagonay (Mh). Therefore different combinations of the E locus alleles, eumelanin inytensifier and eumelanin inhibitors are found in different breeds e.g. Rhodes Island Red has ey/ey Co/? db+/db+ Mh/Mh and New Hampshire has eWh/eWh Co/Co db+/db+ Mh/?. Distribution of eumelanin within individual father results in several type of secondary feather pattern such as barring, spangling, mottling etc. Majority of the secondary plumage pattern have autosomal inheritance such as stippling (Pg), lacing (La), autosomal barring (Ab) etc and found to show incomplete dominance. Hence secondary plumage pattern are due to interactions of secondary as well as primary plumage genes e.g. for Stipping secondary plumage pattern, e+, pg+ , Co+, db+, ml+, Mo+. Apart from autosomal inherited secondary plumage pattern, some secondary plumage patter are sex linked such as sex linked barring.

Investigations on genetic basis of beautiful and uniform plumage colour patterns of guinea fowl were initiated by Italian geneticist Dr. Alexandro Ghigi (Ghigi 1924, 1966). His reports presented at the 2nd World's Poultry Congress, Barcelona, and Subsequently at the 13th World's Poultry Congress, Kier described identification of nine distinct plumage phenotypes. Genetic determination was suggested through the genes segregating at three independent loci, 2 with recessive alleles and one with incompletely dominant alleles. Subsequently these findings were also confirmed by Greenwood (1987). Another independent study conducted at the University of Connecticut, by Somes (1990, 1996) presented evidence for existence of a fourth autosomal "Dundoite" (D/d) locus to explain the inheritance of chamois plumage colour. His reports described existence of at least 17 different plumage colour patterns including those indentified in the earlier literature and other sources (Ghigi 1924, 1966, Van-Hoesen and Stromberg 1975, Greenwood 1987). In all these investigations, the ancestral plumage colour pattern of wild helmeted guinea fowl characterized with evenly distributed white spots or 'pearls' on dark-grey or violet-black background colour was adopted as the 'wild type' standard or normal phenotype. It is against this plumage colour that the inheritance of all identified mutants was compared.

i. **Margarogene locus (m, M+):** This biallelic autosomal locus determine the 'wild phenotype. Presence of dominant allele 'M' ensure production of feathers of dark-grey or violet-black colour with pearl markings. The 'M' gene also restrict pigment formation to produce pearl appearance. The presence of recessive allele'm' inhibits the formation of pearl markings and production of feathers with solid colour e.g. violet, sky-blue (coral-blue), opline phenotypes etc.

ii. **White colour locus (W, W+):** Presence of incompletely dominant, autosomal 'W' allele inhibits the production of all pigment on ventral body surface and results in a luxedo or varigated phenotype while the dorsal surface show the normal coloured feathers determined by colour genes. Individuals worth homozygous genotype (WW) produce birds of completely white plumage colour.

iii. **Pigment intensity locus (il+):** Presence of 'recessive' 'I' gene cause dilution of dark-grey (wild) colour to sky blue. Alleles at this locus possibly affect the feather structure and thereby bring about the changed plumage colour. The 'I' genes is also epistatic to the dundotte gene, thus birds with homozygous 'ii' genotype show several shades of blue (gray) colourations.

iv. **Dundotte locus (D+d):** Presence of 'recessive gene (d)' produce basic buff-dun background while 'D' allele produce blue colour. But wide variations in the colour intensity may be observed when combined with I+/ I+ genotypes e.g. Dun-buff-iidd, Iidd; Blue-dnn-ii, dd; Blue ii DD, iiDd Possibly, the presence of I'/I and I+I genotyps is some way also inhibit production of eumelanin the dark black pigment characteristic of both M+/M+ and m'/m genotypes. But 'd' gene act differently in presence of 'I'I' genotype which suggest existence of epistasis and production of blue colour.

Somes (1996) observed that the blue plumage colour production in guinea fowl was much clearer and brighter. This shining blue colour is possibly caused by some structural changes in feather. Presence of tiny melanin particles in cells of the horny keratinous outer layer of feather branches perhaps alter the scattering or diffusion of light components and cause production of the shining blue colour. But dark plumage colourations in case of both pearl and royal purple phenotypes were due to more densely packed melanin particles in centre. The action of dun gene would then to be to remove the densely packed melanin particles from the centre of the feather branches. In the case of blue phenotype, the colour would change to a pale-blue colour.

The 'Extender' locus (E-locus) influences on distribution of pigment throughout the plumage has been studied extensively in domestic fowl. Using the E-locus model of fowl, Singh and Singh (1988) and Pal (1992) explained the genetic determination of plumage in guinea fowl. A direct correlation was found between the down colour mutants of the baby keets and adult plumage colourations (Fig 4.1). The most common down feather phenotype, the `wild' type which subsequently develop into the pearl plumage, is characterized by a dorsal median dark brown broad stripe running from head downwards. Laterally on its either side are the yellowish brown and dark brown stripes extending from pygostyle to the base of wings; the remaining area is covered by light brownish down coat. All other down colour phenotypes perhaps represent the dilution of the `wild' colour to light gray or lavender and white. Somes (1992) however observed that these results were obtained because 'dd' genotype was perhaps absent in these stocks.

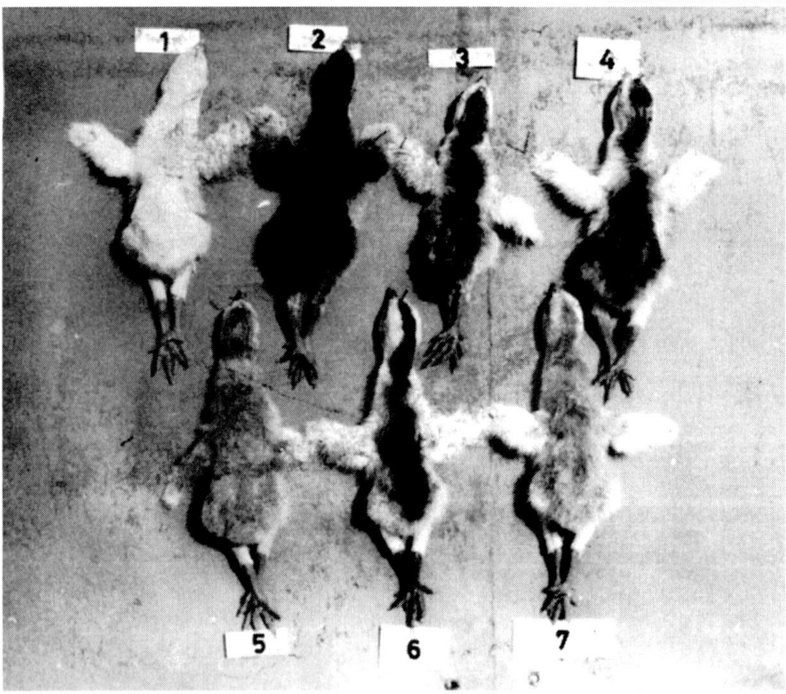

Fig. 4.1 : Down plumage colouration among keets. Left to Right: 1: White, 2: Pearl, 3: Violet, 4: Pearl White Breasted, 5: Lavender, 6: Violet white breasted, 7: Lavender white breasted

The results of plumage colour segregations among the progeny obtained from different matings (Table 4.1) showed all white progeny from the matings among white parents and coloured keets only from the matings between coloured parents. It indicate existence of an autosomal pigment gene 'C' essential for all melanophore activities. These mating studies further suggest dominance of pearl over lavender and white; and lavender over white. It is proposed that the intensity of melanin in down and adult plumage is determined through the E-locus alleles viz. e+ (dark gray); el (lavender) and e (white). Thus these alleles show a decreasing order of dominance at the E (extended self black) locus. The appearance of lavender keets obtained from the matings involving pearl parents and the testcross mating at 10 and 15 support the existence of this triple allelic series (Table 4.2).

Secondary colour pattern gene (s) regulates the distribution of pigment within each individual feather as observed in case of the spotting and splashing pattern. Matings 3, 8 and 12 suggest that spotting was observed only when a dominant autosomal spotting gene (Sp) was inherited. A third independent locus determined the splashing or restriction of colour

in White breasted varieties. The splashing gene$_s$ (S) was dominant over its absence as evident in mating at sr. no. 10, 11, 12 and 17 in table 4.1 (Singh and Singh, 1988).

Table 4.1 : Segregation of plumage colour phenotype during the matings between varieties. PP: Pearl, LL: Lavender, VV: Violet, WW: White, PWB: Pearl white breasted, LWB: lavender white breasted

S. No	Type of mating (SirexDam)	Plumage colour of offsprings						
		PP	LL	VV	WW	PWB	LWB	Total
Matings within plumage colours								
1	PP x PP	2088	52	-	-	-	-	2140
2	LL x LL	-	1858	-	-	-	-	1858
3	VV x VV	-	-	189	-	-	-	189
4	WW x WW	-	-	-	760	-	-	760
Matings between plumage colours								
5	PWB x WW	34	3	-	41	124	6	208
6	LWB x LWB	-	20	-	1	-	19	40
7	PP x LL	290	58	-	-	56	5	309
8	LL x PP	277	24	-	-	22	5	338
9	PP x VV	3	3	-	-	-	-	6
10	PP x WW	-	-	-	18	204	24	246
11	LL x PWB	3	10	-	-	13	4	30
12	PWB x LL	3	3	-	-	12	3	21
13	VV x PWB	9	3	-	-	6	-	18
Test-crosses matings								
14	WW x PP	106	3	-	-	325	37	471
15	WW x LL	-	61	-	-	230	107	398

16	LL x WW	-	3	-	27	174	55	259
17	WW x VV	-	2	-	-	48	-	50
18	VV x WW	-	-	-	2	12	1	15
19	WW x PWB	2	8	19	-	37	-	66
20	WW x LWB	-	5	-	9	-	23	37

Table 4.2 : Major genes affecting plumage colour in guinea fowl

S. No	Locus and plumage trait	Gene Symbol	Description
1	C-Locus-two alleles for colour manifestation	C	Presence of pigment
		c	Complete absence of pigment
2	E-Locus- multiple alleles for productionof self extended grades of black colour throughout the plumage of both sexes in presence of dominant `C' allele	E	Production of self extended black pigment
	i. Pearl (wild mutant)	e^+	Production of self extended dark grey pigment; dominant over e^l and e.
	ii. Lavender (liliac mutant)	e^l	Dilution of the dark grey pigment throughout the plumage; dominant over e
	iii. White (recessive mutant)	e	Complete failure of pigment production in homozygotes.
3	S-Locus-two alleles for splashing of white colour	S	Failure of pigment formation in breast feathers. Complete dominance.

		s	No splashing (solid colour
4	Sp-Locus-two alleles for spotting or restriction of pigment formation	Sp	Restricted pigmentation (spotting) of all adult feathers. Complete dominance.
		sp	No spots (solid colouration)

Feather development genes

At hatching time each keet is completely covered with down feathers. Subsequent replacements by contours, juvenile and adult plumage is gradual and takes place in a very orderly manner essentially similar to that observed in domestic fowl. During these events newly hatched keets may be characterized as slow feathering and rapid feathering on the basis of primary wing feather development. Micek and Malik (1970) identified significant differences in remige length between male and females at 4, 8 and 12 days of age. Based on these observations genetic control through sex-linked locus was suggested.

Plumage studies of day old keets established existence of two distinct flight feather mutant phenotypes namely rapid feathering and slow feathering keets (Fig 4.2). In rapid feathering keets the coverts are of about same length as that of the primary feathers while in slow feathering keets these feathers are only about two-third as long and also more slender. Detailed observations showed that about 84% keets revealed correct phenotype at day old stage. Among the doubtful phenotypes at day old stage, about 9% could be corrected by further confirmations at 4th day and 10th day when these differences became more prominent. Rapid feathering keets also reveal much better developed tail feathers (Fig 4.2).

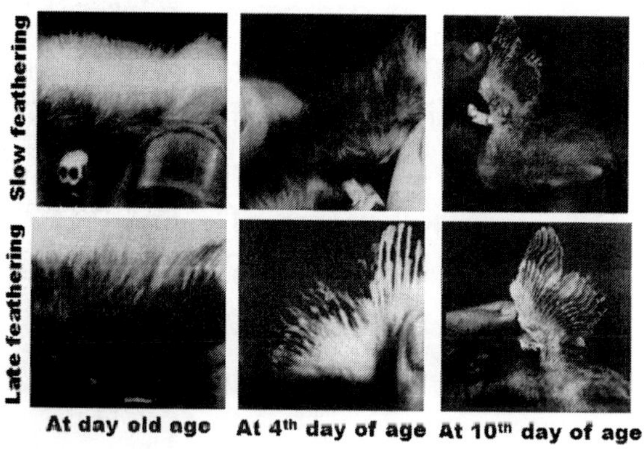

Fig. 4.2 : Slow and rapid feathering in guinea fowl at different ages

Inheritance investigations with progeny from parents of known feathering phenotypes indicate genetic control through sex linked biallelic (K, k+) locus for this trait, where 'rapid' feathering was the recessive phenotype (Table 4.3). Dosage effects were also identified in slow feathering male keets which show very poor development of primary feathers. Inheritance data further indicated possible existence of some other background genes which influenced this trait. Nearly 6-7% progeny showed discrepancy in determination of correct feathering phenotype.

Table 4.3 : Expected and observed frequencies of slow and rapid feathering progenies from the matings between slow and rapid feathering parents

Mating Type (Sire x Dam)	N	Expected phenotype				Observed phenotype			
		Male		Female		Male		Female	
		SF	RF	SF	RF	SF	RF	SF	RF
KK (SF) x K(SF)	27	13.5	-	13.5	-	15	-	12	-
KK (SF) x K^+(RF)	36	18.8	-	18.0	-	20	-	16	-
Kk (SF) x K(SF)	63	31.7	-	15.7	15.7	28	-	18	17
Kk^+ (SF) x K^+(RF)	63	15.7	15.7	15.7	15.7	20	17	12	14
k^+k^+ (RF) x K(SF)	44	22	-	-	22	20	-	-	24
K^+K^+ (RF) x K^+(RF)	26	-	13	-	13	-	15	-	11

(N: Number of progenies)

The distribution of slow and rapid phenotypes was not significantly different among the three varieties; but significantly higher frequency of occurrence for rapid feathering phenotype was observed among the population not selected for growth traits. Attempts to develop rapid feathering (k+/k+)

male and slow feathering (K) female parent lines for auto-sexing of keets at hatch may likely to be successful in case of guinea fowl; since feathering locus in this species is not associated with ev-locus (endogenous viral infection) which is responsible for reduced egg production and higher mortality among the progeny of slow feathering domestic fowl females.

The identification of sex-linked locus responsible for the timing of feather development in three domestic galliform species viz. domestic fowl, turkey and guinea fowl is certainly of great interest for students of comparative genetic aspects. Even though no such situation has been reported in quail and pheasants etc. but present observations suggest that feather development related DNA may be conserved on the Z chromosome in this order of bird (Pal and Singh, 1997a).

Variants of axial skeleton

Existence of at least two axial skeleton variants was recorded in two apparently healthy females of Pearl variety of first generation. Although no inheritance investigations were carried out, but both conditions seem to be inherited through recessive gene at two different loci.

Approtopteria or 'Penguin' guinea fowl : This phenotype was identified by absence of flight feathers and tail feathers. Existence of this condition in guinea fowl has been reported earlier also. It is inherited through an autosomal recessive gene.

Crooked keel : Instead of an usual straight and pointed keel bone, one female bird revealed existence of relatively much short 'Y' shape keel bone. This bird also showed specific weakness of the sternum. A similar skeletal variant is already identified in chicken; its inheritance was hypothesized through an autosomal recessive gene. Present observation is the first report regarding the existence of the 'crooked keel' condition in guinea fowl.

Helmet form : Existence of bi-lobed or M shaped helmet form has been observed in a few male guinea fowl individuals. Preliminary observations indicated inheritance through a simple autosomal recessive gene; although hormonal influences could not rule out. Since mode of inheritance was not definitely ascertained, apparently it needs further confirmation.

B. Biochemical Polymorphism

Inherited differences among individuals or genetic polymorphism refers to existence of two or more than two alternative hereditary forms that can be easily distinguished from each other and whose inheritance is simple Mendelian in nature.

Existence of large number of qualitative variations of body proteins, enzymes, and alloantigen molecules defined by immunological, electrophoretic and biochemical approaches have been reported for farm bred avian species. These simple polymorphic traits are controlled by Mendalian genes and their loci are distributed throughout the genome. Accurately determined, these characters are not influenced by environment and these remain unchanged throughout the lifespan. The primary functions of these molecule are not fully understood. In fact the polymorphic systems constitute an ideal source of fairly neutral marker genes. The higher amenability of these marker genes to deductive analysis has yielded interesting information regarding genetic organisation, population structure, genetic distances between populations, and phylogenetic relations. Although their existence and biological significance remains a true puzzle of biology but several studies have established apparent relationship of these polymorphic genes to survivability and fitness traits. Significant association of marker gene have also been demonstrated with economic traits e.g. fertility, survival, productivity or disease resistance.

Table 4.4 Biochemical polymorphisms in avian species

Polymorphic systems	Guinea fowl	Domestic fowl
A. Biochemical systems:		
Blood proteins	2	7
Egg white proteins	3	8
Enzymes		>27
B. Immunological systems:		
Blood groups	8(?)	13
Agglutinogens	1	>18
Lymphocytes alloantigens	-	-
Allotypes G1	-	14

Immunogenetic variations

Inherited differences among individuals or genetic polymorphisms when studied by immunological methods are immunogenetic variants. Blood groups are of fundamental importance to immunogenetics but variations have also been identified for alloantigens of lymphocytes, immunoglobulin allotypes, euglobulins, lipoproteins etc. These aspects have been studied in more details in case of chicken, existence of 13 blood group systems determined through 13 different autosomal loci and immunoglobulins allotypes are established.

Blood group polymorphism: Heritable erythrocytic antigenic variations, identified by serological methods are referred as blood groups. Alloantiserum (blood typing reagents) for identification of blood groups antigens is obtained by selective adsorptions from iso-immune raised in inbred lines and rarely hetero-immunesera. Specific blood group reagents contain only one population of antibodies. A blood group system includes all the antigens which are determined by different gene that behave as though they were controlled through one locus. Blood group system may be simple or complex consisting of a few or several antigenic specificities respectively. Although a potent method of genetic analysis, but the gene-antigen relationship may be considered degenerate in nature since the actual antigenic specificities are far removed from the specific gene controlling it. Due to the inherent difficulties and cost involved in development of blood group reagents only limited headway was made in identification of erythrocytic or leucocytic antigens of guinea fowl. Our knowledge of the guinea fowl blood groups is still very fragmentary. Preliminary investigations using iso-immune and hetero-immune sera and also lecteins of plant and animal origin indicated existence of several simple blood group specificities. Bushchinwilli (1962) successfully isolated 12 mono specific immunesera corresponding erythrocytic antigenic specificities designated as Ea-D, Ea-E, Ea-F, Ea-G, Ea-H, Ea-I, Ea-J and Ea-K. Inheritance investigations indicated genetic control through independent autosomal loci, dominant allele determined the presence of antigen while recessive controlled its absence. In another independent investigation, Shirashi et al., (1978, 1979) reported low incidence of an agglutinegen "Gf" in four guinea fowl strains. Inheritance studies indicated determination through a dominant autosomal gene. Further investigations with numigal (guinea fowl X chicken) hybrids showed that the Gf alloantigen could be serolgically classified into Gf1 and Gf2 subtypes, while former was detected in both genetic group but Gf1 was observed only in guinea fowl. Similarly, existence of two antigens (1z1, 1z2) was reported in guinea fowl (Singh, 1998). Parentage determination through polyvalent antisera showed limited success perhaps due to limited antigenic variability of guinea fowl red cells.

Agglutionogens: Plant lecteins are glycoproteins that may non-covalently bind many species carbohydrates groups present on red cell surface and cause agglutination. Lectein are known to act as valuable probes for identification of individual differences in red cell agglutinability. These natural haemogglinins have attained distinct importance due to their wide applicability to problems in immunobiology and also in clinical pathology. Genetic determination has been reported for presence of several such agglutinogens in poultry species. Testing of guinea fowl red cells with 28 different lecteins revealed distinct individual variations in agglutination reactions Testing of red cells with phytogglutinin from Anacardium occidentale, Anthocephalus uticus, Bauhinia purpurea, Bischofia javanica, Cassia javanica, Semeperuirens, Livistona chinensia, Plerospermum acerifolicum revealed distinct strong agglutination reaction in 2-60 % individuals, while all other lecteins should positive reaction in case of all the sample. But inheritance studies failed to indicate genetic control (Singh et al. 1995).

JEV-Agglutinogen: Another study with Japanese encephalitis virus (JEV) revealed distinct agglutination reaction with guinea fowl erythrocytes. Although age related variations were observed in reactivity but adult birds always showed consistent reactivity levels. Thus three distinct phenotypes: high, low or negative were observed. Preliminary inheritance studies indicated Mendelian inheritance where dominant allele determined the high titre group (Singh *et al.* 1995).

Isoenzyme polymorphism

Biochemical and physiological studies have established genetic variations for several proteins and enzymes in poultry species. The term 'isozyme' refer to all physically distinct multiple enzyme forms with same catalytic actions. Both qualitative and quantitative differences constitute gene determined polymorphisms of proteins or enzyme components. Existence of interesting polymorphisms have been reported for body proteins, enzymes and related biochemical entities for different poultry species. Most of these variations were identified using different biophysical and biochemical techniques particularly electrophoretic methods. Different proteins have different electrical charges. When placed in an appropriate buffer solution and subjected to an electrical potential these migrate towards the anode or the cathode, depending upon their charge. Their rate of migration is influenced by the intensity of their electrical charge and by molecular size and shape. After electrophoresis and appropriate staining using histochemical techniques these proteins are identified as bands in the starch-gel, agar gel or any other medium in which buffer solution is held. Hitherto investigations show that guinea fowl harbor relatively lower level of genetic variations vis a vis domestic fowl.

Table 4.5 Polymorphic status of some proteins in guinea fowl and chicken

Polymorphic system	inheritance	Guinea fowl	Domestic fowl
Haemoglobin (Hb)	A, CD	Monomorphic	Polymorphic (3)
Serum albumin (Alb)	A, CD	Polymorphic (2)	Polymorphic (3)
Serum transferrins (Tf)	A, CD	Polymorphic (3)	Polymorphic (3)
Ovalbumin (Ov)	A, CD	Polymorphic (2)	Polymorphic (2)
G2 ovoglobulin (G2)	A, CD	Polymorphic (2)	Polymorphic (>2)
G3 ovoglobulin (G3)	A, CD	Polymorphic (2)	Polymorphic (>7)
Ovomacroglobulin (Omg)	A, CD	Polymorphic (2)	Polymorphic (2)

Note: A: Autosomal inheritance; CD: Co-dominant inheritance. Figures in parenthesis indicate number of alleles reported).

Serum albumin - Alb : Genetic heterogeneity for this most abundant serum protein was established by Shiraishi et al. (1978). Existence of three distinct albumin

phenotypes viz. AA, BB and AB controlled by two co-dominant autosomal alleles AlbA and AlbB was also confirmed later (Singh and Singh, 1988 and Pal and Singh, 1992).

Transferrin (Conalbumin) - Tf : Transferrins are iron binding glycoproteins present in body fluids. Three electrophoretic variants each consisting of two bands have been observed in diversified guinea fowl populations (Croizier 1967, Kierek-Jaszczuk 1976, Casuka 1979, Singh and Singh 1988). Genetic determination through three autosomal alleles have been reported (Pal and Singh, 1992).

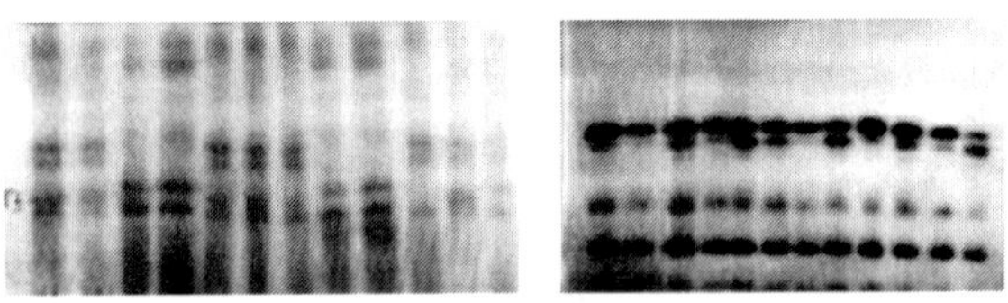

Fig. 4.3 : Electrophoresis pattern showing polymorphism in serum tranferrin (Left) and ovalbumin (Right)

Ovalbumin - Ov : During electrophoresis, this major egg-white protein separate out as intensely staining three anodal bands of diminishing mobility. Existence of two ovalbumin variants are reported, and Ov-A was relatively faster and more predominant variant in all the investigated populations (Casuka

1979, Singh and Singh 1988; Pal and Singh 1992). Inheritance studies revealed genetic control through two co-dominant alleles.

Ovoglobulin-G : Egg-white ovoglobulins or mucinoglobulins consists of three distinct electrophoretic components. The slowest G1 component is the lysozyme which separate towards cathod. Polymorphism has been reported for the ovoglobulin G2 and G3 components. The G2 fraction migrate just behind the G3 fraction. Valenta and Mikolasek (1971) identified two ovoglubulin G2 electrophonetic variants in three phenotypic combinations. Similar variants with three phenotypes were also observed for ovoglobulin G3.

Haemoglobin (HB): As in case of other galliforms birds, guinea fowl haemoglobin (Hb) resolve into two electrophoretic components viz. Hb-M and Hb-m but individual variants were not observed (Hilgert and Vogtiskove 1959, Singh and Singh 1988). Existence of guinea fowl embryonic haemoglobin components have been described by Pal and Singh (1994).

Serum Amlylase - Am (EC-3.2.1) : Avian plasma contains sufficiently high levels of á-amylases. Existence of three amylase variants in five phenotypic combinations was reported (Pal and Singh, 1992). Genetic control was suggested through three co-dominant alleles.

Mannosephosphate isomerase: Mip I : Shiraishi and Hirai (1983) established presence of genetic variants for liver and pancreas mannosephosphate isomerase. Three phenotyps determined by two autosomal alleies viz. MpilA and MpilB were reported.

Cytoplasmic aconitase (Cytosolic aconitase or AconB): Electrophoretic studies revealed monomorphic band B for guinea fowl C to plasmic aconitace from liver. But its electrophoretic pattern was different and anodal than that of chicken. In case of numigal hybrids both variants were observed, but presence of only one variant suggest involvement of sex linked locus (Baverstock et al. 1982). Male hybrids revealed double band pattern (AconA/ AconB) while female showed only A conA type. Results confirmed sex linkage in this. But not exhibit compensation in case of homozygotes. vis a vis heterozygotes (Females). Although individual variations were not observed but distinct electrophoretic heterogenetly was observed in case of alkaline phosphatase Akp-I and Akp-II (3.1.31), glyoxalase (4.4.15), esterase-D (3.1.1) and lysozyme ly (3.2.1.17) (Pal and Singh 1992).

Table 4.6 : Variability of some enzymes in guinea fowl

Enzyme	Gene action	Guinea fowl	Domestic fowl
Adenylaze kinase (2.7.4.3)	A, CD	Monomorphic	Monomorphic
Phosphogluco mutase (2.7.51)	A, CD	Monomorphic	Polymorphic
Esterase - D (Es) (3.1.1.1)	A, CD	Monomorphic	Monomorphic
Alkaline phosphatase - I (Akp) (3.1.3.1)	A, CD	Polymorphic	Polymorphic
Alkaline phosphatase-II (Akp) (3.1.3.1)	A, CD	Polymorphic	Polymorphic
Amylase - I (Am) (3.2.1.1)	A, CD	Polymorphic	Polymorphic
Lysozyme (3.2.1.17)	A, CD	Monomorphic	Polymorphic
Adenosine deaminase (Ad) (3.5.4.4)	A, CD	Monomorphic	Polymorphic
Cytoplasmic aconitase (Acon)	SL	Monomorphic	Monomorphic

Note: A: Autosomal inheritance; SL: Sex-linked inheritance; CD: Co-dominant inheritance. Figures in parenthesis indicate number of alleles reported).

Gene frequencies of biochemical systems were used to estimate the level of genetic variations existing in guinea fowl vis-à-vis chicken. Observations on the proportion of polymorphic (P) and mean heterozygosity H are oddly at variance with respect to results for other

farm-bred avian species. The observed values in case of guinea fowl are significantly lower than the corresponding estimates reported for chicken and quails (Pal 1992). But considering the enzyme heterogeneity level and enzyme functions, the presently observed variations for the regulatory, non-regulatory and variable substrate enzymes of guinea fowl indicate good agreement with respect to variations reported for such enzymes in chicken and quails (Pal 1992).

Table 4.7 : Variability of some enzymes in guinea fowl

Parameters/Gene action	Guinea fowl	Domestic fowl
Number of loci studied	19	19
Number of polymorphic loci	0.6	13
Proportion of polymorphic loci	0.315	0.684
Average heterozygosity	0.032	-

Quantitative variations of enzymes and minerals: existence of gene determined variations has been reported for activity levels of several enzymes and minerals in poultry species. Assay of enzyme activities in guinea fowl also showed wide ranging individual variations besides existence of significant age, sex and varietal effects. Identification of gene effects is always difficult in case of all such traits where quantitative phenotype may be many steps removed from gene products but investigation revealed low to medium heritability values and also indicated significant dominant gene influences besides the additive genetic effects for alkaline phosphatase, amylase, geathione eysozyme and potassium levels in blood (Pal and Singh 1997b; Pal et al. 1996a,b).

Table 4.8 : Heritability values of enzyme activity level

Enzyme	Source	Heritability
Alkaline phosphatase (3.1.3.1)	Serum	0.477±021
Amylase (3.2.1.1)	Serum	0.40±0.015
Lysozyme (3.2.1.17)	Serum	0.311±027
Lysozyme (3.2.1.17)	Egg White	0.770±0.160
Glutathione	RBC	0.521±0.521
Potassium Content	RBC	0.470±0.230
Cholesterol level	Serum	0.340±0.320
High density li protein	Serum	0.320±0.18
Total protein	Serum	0.110± -
Uric acid	Serum	0.390±0.190

❑❑❑

Chapter **5**

Quantitative Genetics

The quantitative genetics can be defined as the study of inheritance of traits, which show continuous variation and are governed by number of traits. These traits are called as quantitative traits as they can be quantified. Some of them are called metric traits as they are measurable on some metric scale e.g. body weight in g and shank length in cm. Some traits are measured in terms of counting such as number of eggs laid during some specified period. Some quantitative traits come in "all or none" class and have only two values i.e. either present or absent. Such traits are fertility, hatchability and mortality. The inheritance of all the quantitative traits is complex as they are governed by number of genes and these genes may interact with each other in number of ways. Further the phenotypic expressions of these traits are influenced to a varying degree by environment. In chicken, the important quantitative traits are growth rate, egg production traits, feed efficiency trait, carcass traits, meat and egg quality traits as well as reproductive and fitness traits.

Inheritance of Economic traits

The domesticated poultry is reared for economic purposes and the purpose is to get meat or egg or both from the poultry. While the meat is produced through gaining weight by the bird itself (either male or female), eggs are produced by the female birds as a natural phenomenon after getting sexual maturity. Hence there are number of factors which influence the meat and egg production from poultry. Meat and egg production potential is genetically controlled and inherited, however they are also influenced by environment as well as the interaction between genetic potential and the environment. For meat and egg production potential, large variation exists between as well as within the populations, but this variation is of continuous type i.e. no distinct phenotypes exists for these traits (like plumage colour), rather the individuals are distributed in a range of minimum to maximum e.g. body weight at day old age may range from 28 g to 38 g in chicken. The traits showing continuous variation are called quantitative traits. These traits are measurable in term of a quantity e.g. body weight of a chick at day old age is 31.5 g or a bird produced 200 eggs in a year. The quantitative traits are polygeneic in nature, means these traits are under the control of many genes. These genes may interact in an additive or non-additive or in both manners with each other. Further, as stated above these traits are influenced by environment and the interaction between genetic potential and environment. Hence the inheritance of these traits is complex and difficult to measure. These traits are also correlated with each other and this correlation may be positive, as heavier egg from heavier bird or negative, as birds giving more eggs have low egg weight. This co-relationship between the traits is also controlled by genes and influenced by environment. Since the part of the variations existing in the traits and co-variations existing between the traits controlled by genotype is inherited, therefore it is essential to measure it. The measures of estimating the genetic variability and co-variability are known as genetic parameters.

Genetic Parameters

Heritability: The heritability estimates the proportion of the total phenotypic variation that is due to heredity. More precisely, it is the proportion of the differences for that trait in a population that is due to heredity. For example if a trait has a heritability of 0.5, it means that 50 % of the total phenotypic variability observed for that trait is due to genotype, while remaining 50 % is due to environment. Therefore, in general heritability (h^2) is defined as the ratio of genotypic variance and phenotypic variance i.e. V_G/V_P. This is defining the heritability in broad sense. In narrow sense, heritability is the ratio of variance due to additive effect and total phenotypic variance i.e. V_A/V_P. The heritability can also be defined in term of regression coefficient. The regression of progeny means on mid-parent means gives the estimate of heritability.

Genetic correlations: The relationship between two traits in statistical term is expressed by correlation. Genetic correlation between two traits is defined as the correlation between genetic effects that influences the two traits (Falconer, 1960). As the phenotype is considered to be a function of both the genotype and environment, therefore the observable or phenotypic correlation between two traits will arise due to correlations between genetic and environmental effects that influence the two traits. Genetic correlation between two traits may arise due to pleiotropy and linkage (Falconer, 1960). Pleiotropy is simply the property of a gene whereby it affects two or more characters, so that if the gene is segregating it causes simultaneous variation in the characters it affect. The degree of correlation arising from pleiotropy expresses the extent to which two characters are influenced by same genes. But as the correlation resulting from pleiotropy is the overall or net effects of all segregating genes, some gene may tend to increase both characters while other may decrease them, thus pleiotropy does not necessarily cause a detectable correlation. Genetic correlation may also be caused by linkage disequilibrium, which is transient in nature. Genetic correlations may also be caused by different breeding goals within a population (Pirchner, 1983). Genetic correlation, like heritability can be estimated from pair of traits using either variance and covariance components (Snedecor, 1940) or the regression of one trait of offspring on other trait of parents and vice versa (Hazel, 1943). Becker (1986) outlined the procedure of estimating the genetic correlations using analysis of variance and covariance, analogous to estimation of heritability.

Inheritance of Meat Production traits

As the meat is produced through gaining weight by the bird itself, therefore the growth is the most important trait for meat production. The growth can very simply be measured in terms of the body weight at a specific age. Another measure of growth may be weight gain in a given time/ age interval and the weight gain may be either absolute or relative. While the absolute weight gain is the difference in body weight taken at different time of age, the relative weight gain is the increase in weight in proportion to a body weight at a given age. There are other traits also to be considered when meat production is to be taken in total and these traits are the efficiency of the birds to utilize feed efficiently for weight gain, yields of the edible meat and quality of the edible meat. Therefore, following traits are important for meat production.

Growth traits

The growth rate is slow in guinea fowl compared to domestic fowl. Age, sex, variety, season and feed efficiency are the few important factors which significantly affect the growth performance Attempts were made to identify the extent of their influences in guinea fowl. Average body weights at different weeks of age are shown in Table 5.1. The weight gains and relative weight gains during different weeks of age are shown in Table 5.2. Observations with respect to varietal differences in body weights are not consistent.

Table 5.1 : Mean body weights at different weeks of age in guinea fowl varieties.

Varieties	Body weight in g			
	0 d	4th wk	8th wk	12th wk
Pearl	27.94	191.76	578.10	956.63
Lavender	27.48	194.86	571.63	950.03
White	27.29	152.00	497.09	879.83

Table 5.2 : Mean body weights at different weeks of age in guinea fowl varieties

Variety	Different periods of age (in weeks)				
	0-4 wk	5-8 wk	9-12 wk	0-8 wk	0-12 wk
Weight gain in g					
Pearl	163.82	386.34	378.54	550.16	944.63
Lavender	167.38	376.77	378.40	544.15	938.03
White	124.71	345.09	382.75	469.80	867.83
Relative weight gain					
Pearl	586.32	201.47	97.98	1969.07	3380.93
Lavender	609.16	193.35	100.43	1980.36	3413.80
White	457.01	227.04	110.91	1721.66	3180.32

Prediction of body weight: Regression equations developed for prediction of 12 wk body weight on the basis of various combinations of early body weights and conformation traits revealed limited accuracy which ranged between 1.3 to 49.2%. Prediction equations developed on body weights showed higher accuracy compared to conformation traits since genetic and phenotypic correlations among body weights were higher than between body weights and conformation traits. Most optimum equation was:

$$Y = 103.45 + 4.39\,X_1 + 0.84X_2 + 35.35X_3$$

Where Y is the predicted 12 wk body weight in gm, X_1 and X_2 are body weight at day old and 8 wks age in gm and X_3 is 8 wk shank length in cm (Mundra, 1990).

Confirmation traits

The shank length, keel length and breast angle was studied in guinea fowl (Table 5.3). Significant varietal differences were observed for shank length and keel length at 12 wk and 8 wks of age ($P < 0.01$).

Table 5.3 : Mean estimates for confirmation traits at different weeks of age in males and females guinea fowl

Age	Male	Female	CV %
Keel length (cm)			
8 week	6.2 ± 0.04	6.1 ± 0.03	11.4
12 week	8.1 ± 0.05	7.8 ± 0.03	9.9
16 week	9.9 ± 0.44	9.3 ± 0.03	19.4
Shank length (cm)			
8 week	4.7 ± 0.03	4.6 ± 0.02	11.6
12 week	6.4 ± 0.03	6.2 ± 0.02	9.3
16 week	7.3 ± 0.23	6.9 ± 0.02	7.9
Breast angle (º):			
12 week	34.2 ± 0.21	34.1 ± 0.14	10.0
16 week	37.1 ± 0.26	36.5 ± 0.18	7.9

Feed efficiency traits

Estimates for average feed consumption, feed efficiency and gain in body weight for 192 half-sibs of the three varieties belonging to 32 sire families raised from 4 wk to 16 wk of age were obtained on sire mean basis (Singh et al. 1989). Feed efficiency decreased with the advancement of age, most sharp decrease was observed after 12 wk of age (Table 5.4). Feed efficiency ranged from 2.2 to 6.9, it was 4.71 at the age of 10 to 12 wk. Coefficient of variation among sire groups ranged from 9 to 12, 12 to 10 and 12 to 18 percent for feed consumption, feed efficiency and gain in body weight. Results showed existence of significant differences between sires but not between the varieties.

Table 5.4 : Mean feed efficiency traits during different weeks of age in guinea fowl

Traits	Age in weeks			
	4-6	7-8	9-10	11-12
Feed consumed(g)	304.1	560.3	668.6	826.6
Gain in weight(g)	142.0	158.6	175.3	173.8
Feed efficiency	2.2	3.5	3.8	4.8

Carcass traits

Carcass and meat studies of guinea fowl growers of different ages (Table 5.5 and 5.6) revealed best dressing percentage (including giblets) of about 77.0 per cent for 12 wk old birds, a value slightly higher than the commonly

Table 5.5 : Percent carcass and giblet yields and various losses at different weeks of slaughtering in guinea fowl birds

Age wks	Live weight	Carcass weight	Evs. yield %	Giblet yield %	Blood + feather loss %	Offal loss%
12	930.6^{a} ± 16.66	724.52^{a} ±13.72	77.85^{a} ±0.96	6.28^{a} ±0.24	8.29^{a} ±0.58	8.25^{a} ±1.43
16	1224.0^{b} ± 17.37	936.15^{b} ±15.45	76.49^{a} ±0.42	5.88^{a} ±0.17	9.82^{a} ±0.45	7.75^{a} ±0.77
56	1624.3^{c} ± 27.15	1207.3^{c} ±18.74	74.16^{b} ±0.71	4.83^{b} ±0.19	9.37^{a} ±0.50	12.6^{b} ±0.82

Note : Figures bearing the same superscript are not significantly different with each other

Table 5.6 : Percent cut up parts yield at different weeks of slaughtering in guinea fowl birds

Age in weeks	Wing	Drum stick	Thigh	Breast	Back	Neck
12	14.21^{a} ± 0.34	12.97^{a} ± 0.54	16.26^{a} ± 0.37	28.45^{a} ± 0.55	23.63^{a} ± 0.51	6.46^{a} ±0.28
16	13.88^{a} ± 0.15	13.07^{a} ± 0.15	15.24^{b} ± 0.15	27.78^{a} ± 0.17	22.32^{a} ± 0.25	5.71^{a} ±0.16
56	12.71^{b} ± 0.33	12.49^{a} ± 0.21	14.35^{c} ± 0.28	27.82^{a} ± 0.57	26.75^{b} ± 0.34	5.86^{a} ±0.18

Note : Figures bearing the same superscript are not significantly different with each other

reported estimates for broilers (Sharma et al., 2000). In well finished birds, breast is wide and dimpled with a good breadth of meat. Most flesh is found on breast (29.9 percent), thighs and drumsticks (25.5%), these cut up parts together account for more than one half of the

total meat. Average meat to bone ratio for cooked carcass was 1.77. These observations further substantiate that 12 wk age was the ideal age for slaughter (market age).

Genetic Parameters of Growth traits

Heritability

Body weight and confirmation traits: Paternal half-sib heritability estimates for the body weight at different ages ranged from 0.28 to 0.76; the highest values were obtained for 0 wk and lowest for 12 wk body weights (Table 5.7). In view of small population Mundra et al., (1993) used BLUP model to get unbiased genetic estimates to get unbiased genetic estimates. Conformation traits showed relatively lower estimates of heritability at all ages (Table 5.8).

Table 5.7 : Heritability estimates for early body weight in guinea fowl

Trait	h^2 estimate	Reference
Body weight at 0 wk	0.32 ± 0.10 to 0.58 ± 0.19	Singh et al. (1988)a, Singh et al. (1991), Mundra et al. (1993)
Body weight at 4 wk	0.26 ± 0.09 to 0.51 ± 0.11	Singh et al. (1988a), Singh et al. (1991), Mundra et al. (1993)
Body weight at 8 wk	0.28 ± 0.10 to 0.53 ± 0.13	Singh et al. (1988a), Singh et al. (1991), Mundra et al. (1993)
Body weight at 12 wk	0.23 ± 0.14 to 0.52 ± 0.13	Singh et al. (1988a), Singh et al. (1991), Mundra et al. (1993)

Guinea fowl has a reputation for preferential mating, therefore, heritability estimates were also assessed from sire components of variance duly adjusted for full-sib relationships after the methods suggested by Bohren (1975). These results revealed that heritability obtained from half-sib correlation method ignoring the higher contributions of dams lead to higher estimates and need to be adjusted for full-sib relationships.

Table 5.8 : Heritability estimates for early body weight in guinea fowl

Traits	Sire families		Reference
12 wk Shank length	44	0.33 ±0.12	Singh et al., 1988b
12 wk Keel length	44	0.37 ± 0.13	
12 wk Breast angle	44	0.42 ± 0.18	
12 wk Shank length	116	0.34 ± 0.19	Mundra et al., 1993
12 wk Keel length	116	0.32 ± 0.20	
12 wk Breast angle	116	0.23 ± 0.13	

Carcass and meat traits: Half-sib analysis of the data for dressing percentage and cut-up parts corrected for significant sex effects revealed low to moderate heritability estimates which ranged between 0.11 to 0.35. Carcass traits and cut-up part values showed moderate

to high phenotypic correlations (rP) while genetic correlations (rG) were relatively low. These estimates are based on small population size; hence need further confirmation with sufficiently large data.

Genetic correlations

Estimates for genetic and phenotypic correlations between body weights and between conformation traits at different ages showed high and positive values (Table 5.9 to 5.11). Similar trends were also observed for these correlations during all subsequent studies. The differences observed in various estimates of genetic parameters could be due to length of prior selection, differences in selection environment and other well known factors. Present results identified polygenic determination for growth traits in guinea fowl and the components of variation were most likely similar to chicken.

Table 5.9 : Genetic correlation between body weight at different ages

Body weight	0 wk BW	4 wk BW	8 wk BW	12 wk BW
0 wk BW	-	0.36±0.21	0.36±0.22	0.37±0.22
4 wk BW		-	0.86±0.07	0.78±0.11
8 wk BW			-	0.92±0.04
12 wk BW				-

Table 5.10 : Genetic correlation between body weights and confirmation traits

Body weight	Conformation traits							
	8th wk SL	8th wk KL	12th wk SL	12th wk KL	12th wk BA	16th wk SL	16th wk KL	16th wk BA
0 wk	0.44± 0.25	0.47± 0.24	0.37± 0.26	0.46± 0.25	0.36± 0.29	0.32± 0.27	0.21± 0.77	0.37± 0.27
4th wk	0.78± 0.12	0.79± 0.12	0.74± 0.14	0.75± 0.15	0.69± 0.19	0.58± 0.21	0.26± 0.79	056± 0.23
8th wk	0.89± 0.07	0.91± 0.06	0.83± 0.10	0.82± 0.12	0.70± 0.19	0.69± 0.17	0.31± 0.80	0.64± 0.20
12th wk	0.78± 0.13	0.89± 0.07	0.87± 0.08	0.89± 0.07	0.79± 0.14	0.75± 0.15	0.37± 0.78	0.76± 0.15
16th wk	0.72± 0.15	0.83± 0.11	0.86± 0.09	0.87± 0.08	0.77± 0.15	0.79± 0.12	0.39± 0.73	0.82± 0.11

Table 5.11 : Genetic correlation among confirmation traits

Traits	SL-4 wk	KL-8 wk	SL-12 wk	KL-12 wk	BA-12 wk	SL-16 wk	KL-16 wk	BA-12 wk
SL-4 wk	-	0.84± 0.12	0.85± 0.11	0.74± 0.19	0.56± 0.30	0.65± 0.22	0.26± 0.99	0.48± 0.48
KL-8 wk	0.76	-	0.80± 0.15	0.86± 0.11	0.71± 0.22	0.66± 0.23	0.34± 0.96	0.63± 0.25
SL-12 wk	0.50	0.49	-	0.85± 0.16	0.70± 0.22	0.18± 0.13	0.29± 0.96	0.66± 0.23
KL-12 wk	0.53	0.49	0.58	-	0.80± 0.17	0.66± 0.23	0.37± 0.96	0.68± 0.23
BA-12 wk	0.46	0.47	0.46	0.59	-	0.65± 0.25	0.33± 1.05	072± 022
SL-16 wk	0.45	0.44	0.41	0.53	0.56	-	0.31± 0.94	0.65± 0.23
KL-16 wk	0.10	0.20	0.07	0.24	0.32	0.50	-	0.37± 0.94
BA-16 wk	0.31	0.28	0.34	0.33	0.26	0.31	0.12	-

Inheritance of Egg production traits

Guinea fowl females produce considerable number of eggs in each laying seasons. Age at first egg (sexual maturity), egg weight and partial egg production as indicator of total number of eggs laid are the traits of importance for development of breeding plans for their improvement.

Sexual maturity: Factors which influence sexual maturity include management, and growth rate. Guinea fowl females attain sexual maturity at relatively late age. Average age at first egg is about 229.1 ± 1.4 days. Investigations showed that selection for gains in body weight, improvements in management, nutrition and health care have effectively reduced the age at first egg.

Seasonality in egg laying: Mating activity as well as egg laying in guinea fowl is triggered primarily by changes in the season. Egg laying in guinea fowl is initiated with increase in day length after winter season (March/April). Egg production decreased as the day length and ambient temperature reduced considerably (September/October) (Table 5.12). Rise in ambient temperature possibly also has some influence on the initiation of egg production. About 16 to 20% hens also show higher incidence of extended pause period during the peak summer, but little thermal stress was evident on egg shell formation and its thickness.

Table 5.12 : Percent egg production in different months

Month	Av. Temp. (°C)		% production		
	Max.	Min.	Pearl	Lavender	White
March	27.7	15.5	10.0	11.4	10.5
April	33.9	18.8	13.3	13.0	13.6
May	34.4	25.6	16.2	16.3	17.7
June	32.8	23.0	20.5	20.6	18.0
July	36.0	23.4	19.7	20.0	17.7
August	31.6	21.9	14.3	13.2	16.3
September	31.7	20.7	6.0	5.5	6.2

Egg laying: Although distinctly seasonal layers, the guinea fowl females produce considerable number of eggs in each laying cycle. The eggs laid at commencement of laying are usually small in size but final uniform size and normal weight (egg wt. 41.0 ± 0.23 g, length - 49.2 ± 0.16 mm, width - 37.7 ± 1.12 mm) was attained within the first fortnight. Egg weight slightly increased with age of guinea fowl and relatively with each breeding season. On deep litter average production is around 80-100 eggs and hen housed production is 48.7%.

Mean estimates of total egg production, part egg production (PREN) and related traits are presented in Table 5.13. Hens in cages lay more number of eggs compared to the layers kept on floor.

Table 5.13 : Mean estimates of Egg laying traits in guinea fowl

Genetic group	Age at 1st egg (d)	Egg wt. (g)	Egg No. (in 90 d of laying)	Reference
Pearl	258.4± 5.6	-	45.9± 1.8	Singh & Singh, 1990
Lavender/ Pearl	263.8± 4.3	39.6± 0.3	57.7± 1.2	Singh et al., 1993
Lavender	250.1± 4.9	38.3± 0.7	55.2± 3.1	Pal, 1992
Pearl	260.6± 2.6	37.2± 0.3	47.8± 1.6	Pal, 1992
White	251.5± 4.4	39.1± 0.6	65.0± 2.7	Pal, 1992
Overall	253.9± 2.7	38.2± 0.4	55.4± 1.7	Pal, 1992
Lavender/ pearl/ White	229.1± 1.4	-	56.9± 1.54	Kumar et al., 1997

Internal egg quality in guinea fowl: The internal egg quality was evaluated by measuring egg weight, shell thickness, albumin index, yolk index and haugh unit (Table 5.14). The guinea fowl varieties did not showed significant differences for any of the trait except shell thickness, which was significantly higher in White guinea fowl birds in comparison to other two varieties.

Table 5.14 : Mean internal egg quality in guinea fowl eggs

Var.	Egg weight (g)	Shell thickness (mm)	Albumin index	Yolk index	Haugh Unit
Lavender	41.98^{a} ± 0.40	0.45^{a} ± 0.021	0.087^{a} ± 0.002	0.43^{a} ± 0.004	80.91^{a} ± 0.91
Pearl	41.20^{a} ± 0.37	0.45^{a} ± 0.008	0.088^{a} ± 0.003	0.43^{a} ± 0.003	80.60^{a} ± 0.92
White	42.15^{a} ± 0.35	0.49^{b} ± 0.010	0.089^{a} ± 0.002	0.44^{a} ± 0.003	80.99^{a} ± 0.75

Note : Figures bearing the same superscript are not significantly different with each other

Genetic Parameters of Egg production traits

Heritability

Egg production: Genetic studies revealed moderate to high heritability estimates for age at 1st egg (0.38 to 0.73) and moderate values for egg production (Table 5.15). These observations indicate low additive gene effects and more environmental influences. The heritability estimates for different part record egg production (PREN) traits were moderate (0.42 ± 0.20), and their genetic correlation estimates were high (Table 5.16). Prediction equations for total egg production (TEP) based on age at first egg (AFE) and different part egg production records showed increasing multiple regression (R^2) values with increasing part record lengths. Total egg production (TEP) was best predicted with fairly good accuracy using age at first egg and PREN-48 prediction equation (R^2=78.1 %). The addition of body weight information to these equations did not significantly influence the predictive values.

Egg quality traits: The egg quality traits are important with respect to consumer preferences and market requirements. Guinea fowl eggs are relatively small in size (38-40 g) and brown in colour. Its thick, strong shell of low porosity reduces moisture losses and maintains egg contents relatively more wholesome. Egg quality traits are significantly influenced by factors like age, season, feed and management. Egg quality traits showed moderate to high heritability values. Genetic correlations also revealed similar trend (Table 5.15 and 5.16).

Genetic and Phenotypic correlations

Age at 1st egg showed negative genetic correlations with body weight at sexual maturity, egg weight and egg production (Table 5.17 and 5.18). Although most correlations between egg quality traits and with egg production showed moderate estimates but negative values were obtained for correlations between Haugh unit score, egg weight and shell weight.

Table 5.15 : Mean estimates and heritability of annual and part period egg production in guinea fowl

Traits	Mean Values	Sire families	h^2	Reference
Age at 1st egg (egg)	229.1± 1.4	15	0.38± 0.25	Kumar et al ., 1997
Total egg Production	92.8± 1.9	57	0.43± 0.13	Singh et al., 1993
-do-	96.4± 4.6	15	0.63± 0.31	Kumar et al ., 1997
Part record egg Production				
up to 90 d	57.6± 1.2	15	0.47± 0.18	Kumar et al ., 1997
up to 52 d	78.6± 3.4	15	0.45± 0.27	Kumar et al ., 1997
up to 48 d	60.9± 2.8	15	0.45± 0.27	Kumar et al ., 1997
up to 44 d	42.9± 2.1	15	0.45± 0.27	Kumar et al ., 1997
up to 40 d	26.9± 1.5	15	0.42± 0.26	Kumar et al . , 1997

Table 5.16 : Heritability estimates for different egg quality traits

Quality Trait	h^2_S	h^2_D	h^2_{S+D}
Egg weight (g)	0.2± 0.1	0.2± 0.1	0.2± 0.1
Shape index	0.2± 0.1	0.1± 0.1	0.1± 0.1
Shell thickness (mm)	0.7± 0.2	0.3± 0.2	0.5± 0.1
Shell weight (g)	0.3± 0.2	0.6± 0.2	0.5± 0.1
Shell porosity (pores/cm^2)	0.7± 0.3	0.2± 0.1	0.5± 0.1
Shell membrane thickness (mm)	0.5± 0.2	0.6± 0.2	0.5± 0.1

Albumin height (mm)	-	-	-
Albumin index	0.5± 0.2	0.2± 0.2	0.3± 0.1
Albumin weight (g)	0.1± 0.1	0.1± 0.1	0.1± 0.1
Yolk weight (g)	0.2± 0.2	0.1± 0.1	0.2± 0.1
Yolk colour score	-	-	-
Haugh unit score	0.6± 0.3	0.6± 0.2	0.3± 0.1

Existence of low amount of additive genetic variations suggest distinct need to formulate selection programmes for improvement of production potentials of indigenous germplasm as followed in case of domestic fowl. The genes determining better shell quality in guinea fowl might be of special interest in view of the future possibilities.

Table 5.17 : Phenotypic (above diagonal) and genetic (below diagonal) correlation between egg production traits

Trait	Age at 1st egg	Egg weight (g)	Total egg prod-uction	Egg prod-uction (90 days)	Egg shell thick-ness
Age at 1st egg(d)	-	-0.01	-8.15	0.08	-0.01
Egg weight(g)	-0.41± 0.41	-	0.08	0.11	0.15
Total egg production	-0.21± 0.22	0.33± 0.22	-	0.71	0.04
Egg production (90 d)	0.02± 0.21	0.12± 0.22	0.86± 0.67	-	0.01

Table 5.18 : Genetic correlation between egg production traits and part period egg production

Trait	Part egg record production (PREN) of			
	40 d	44 d	48 d	52 d
Age at 1st egg (AFE)	-0.67± 0.57	-0.43± 0.53	0.17± 051	0.04± 0.49
Body weight (BW)at 16 wk	-010± 0.47	0.07± 0.46	0.03± 0.46	0.15± 0.45
Total egg production(TEP)	0.18± 0.17	0.91 ± 0.10	0.98± 0.04	0.94± 0.06

Selection for Economic traits

Selection can be defined in terms of its observable consequences as the 'non-random differential reproduction of genotype' and may be either natural or intentional. The purpose of intentional selection for a meteric character is to modify its mean, to reduce its variability and to extend its range in one direction. The change in population mean resulting from selection is brought through changes of gene frequencies at the loci that influence the character under selection. The change produced by selection that is of interest to breeder is the change of population mean and may be referred as response to selection. Basically, response to selection is the function of additive genetic variability and intensity of selection, but some other factors such as effect of natural selection, inbreeding etc influence the response to selection.

Selection for meteric characters in livestock including poultry is being done largely for improving the traits of economic importance. Since majority of the traits are production related traits such as growth rate, egg production, hence the selection is on positive side i.e. the individuals having higher estimates for these traits are to be selected. In very few cases such as abdominal fat in poultry, individuals having lower estimates are being selected. Therefore either higher or lower side, the individuals are selected on their individual performance for the trait. This is most simple way of selection and is called as mass selection or individual selection. The effectiveness of this selection depends upon the degree of reliability of the phenotype of the individual to be an measure of the genotype of that individual for the trait being selected. This reliability depends upon the extent of influence of the environment on that trait as we know that the phenotype of an individual (P) is equal to the genotype (G) plus environmental influence (E) i.e. P = G + E. In case, where environmental influence is less, P may be a good indicator of G, but in the traits under large environmental influence, P may not be good indicator of G. Therefore to improve the prediction of G from the P, the information from different sources such as ancestors, sibs or progenies may be considered after giving proportional weightage. Hence the selection may be classified in the following methods depending upon the source of information used.

Individual selection: In this method the individual is selected on the basis of its own performance. It is also called as Mass selection. It is also called as Mass selection.

Pedigree selection: In this method the individual is selected on the basis of its own performance as well as the performance the parents/ grandparents.

Progeny selection: In this method the individual is selected on the basis of it's the performance of its progenies.

Selection based on the performance of the collateral relatives: In this method the individual is selected on the basis of its own performance as well as the performance its collateral relatives such as full sibs or half sibs.

The selection may be done for one two or more than traits at a time. Depending upon the number of traits under selection, the selection methods may be classified as follows.

Tandom selection: In this method one trait is selected at a time. After improving one trait, another trait is improved.

Independent Culling Level: In this method two traits are improved simultaneously by sixing the minimum culling levels for both the traits.

Index method: In this method two or more traits are selected simultaneously through an index, in which due weightage is assigned to each trait.

Selection Studies in Guinea fowl

Since in our country, guinea fowl is being reared as rural poultry farming, the systematic efforts to improve guinea fowl are very few. At central Avian Research Institute, Izatnagar, systematic selection is being carried out for high early body weight.

Genetic Improvement of Guncari germplasm: The nucleus germplasm was obtained from local villages surrounding Allahabad and also from P. A. U., Ludhiana. This stock was random bred for two generation. The base population was obtained from this unselected and heterogeneous population and comprised of a total of 1,086 progenies pertaining to 44 sire families in 1987-1988. From this base population, the three varieties were separated and bred true for the plumage type along with selection for high 12th week body weight.

All the three varieties i.e. Pearl, Lavender and White were continued to be regenerated by selecting 9 sires and 50-60 dams in each varieties, having higher 12th week body weight. Mass selection was used for improvement of 12 week body weight. Each sire was used to mate with 5-6 dams in a single sire mating pens. The mating between close relatives was avoided to keep the inbreeding low.

In 1999-2000, the Pearl variety was regenerated as earlier i.e. under 12th week body weight selection programme, while, in Lavender variety, attempts were started to develop divergent lines for antibody response to SRBC and White variety was regenerated through random mating. While the Pearl was continued to improve for 12th week body weight and the white variety was continued to regenerated under random mating, in Lavender varieties, divergent selection programme was continued for 3 generations i.e. up to 2002-03. In 2003-04, the Lavender variety was also being imposed to 12th week body weight selection and was regenerated subsequently under same system.

Body weight: The body weights at different weeks of age in all the three varieties of guinea fowl during this period have been presented in Fig 5.1. Though the body weights at different weeks of age showed wide fluctuations over generation, but an overall increasing trend is quite evident in all the body weights (Sharma and Singh, 2006, Sharma, 2009).

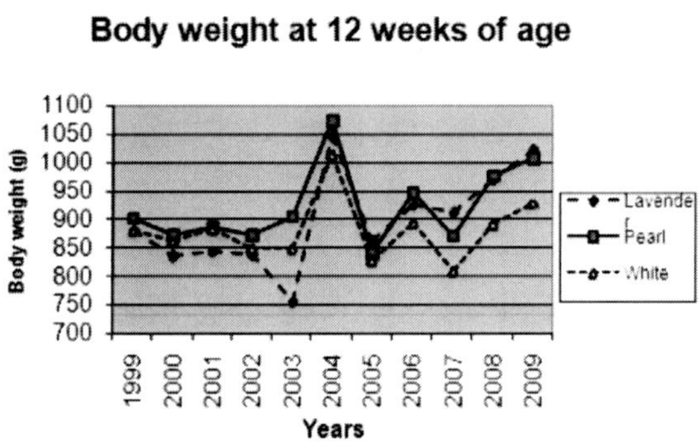

Fig. 5.1 : Body weight at 12th week in three varieties of guinea fowl over generations

Crossbreeding experiment

By definition, cross breeding is the crossing between two well defined breeds. In poultry, cross breeding has a long history. All the assailable chicken commercial germplasm, either of meat type or egg type are the crosses of two or more breeds. Cross breeding, not only give the advantage of hybrid vigour, but also allow combining the advantageous characteristics of two breeds into one. In cross breeding, two effects are important and they are heterosis and reciprocal effects. Heterosis is defined as the deviation of the progenies mean from the mid parent value. Two basic mechanisms, namely dominance and epistasis have been proposed to be responsible for heterosis. Reciprocal effects are the differences between the progenies means produced by using the parents in a combination as well as in reciprocal combination. In chicken, the cross breeding is very well established and there is no dearth of literature on it, however in guinea fowl, very limited information are available. Some information on crossbreeding parameters is presented drom a diallele experiment in guinea fowl (Kumar et al., 1995).

The diallel crosses provide information regarding genetic interactions and maternal and sex-linked effects. These investigations further help in the identification of suitable mating systems based on specific and general combining abilities of the genetic groups. Results of a full diallei mating experiment between the three varieties of guinea fowl viz. Pearl, Lavender and White confirmed that both additive as well as non-additive gene effects were important for body weights and conformation traits. Although purebreds were not significantly different among themselves with respect to body weights (Table 5.19) but their crosses revealed an overall superiority for 12 wk body weight and positive heterosis ranging from 4.5 to 13.0% (Table 5.20). The maximum heterosis and heaviest body weight at 12 wk was obtained for the F1 crosses and reciprocals of Lavender and White parents. Good nicking ability was also observed for shank length at 12 wk, though the magnitude of heterosis was low.

Table 5.19 : Mean estimates for body weight and confirmation traits at different weeks of age in all possible genetic groups under a full di-allele mating

Genetic groups	Body eight (g) at		Shank length (cm) at		Keel length (cm) at	
(Sire x Dam)	8th wk	12th wk	8th wk	12th wk	8th wk	12th wk
Purebreds						
LL x LL	534.38^{a}	822.63^{d}	5.57^{a}	6.63^{b}	7.17^{b}	8.82^{a}
	± 8.45	± 11.26	± 0.04	± 0.05	± 0.05	± 0.08
PP x PP	439.31^{e}	832.48^{cd}	5.55^{a}	6.40^{cd}	6.92^{ab}	8.62^{abc}
	± 11.80	± 19.21	± 0.05	± 0.06	± 0.07	± 0.10
WW x WW	510.70^{ab}	824.78^{d}	5.51^{a}	6.63^{b}	7.08^{a}	8.73^{ab}
	± 4.83	± 7.93	± 0.02	± 0.03	± 0.03	± 0.04
Crossbreds						
LL x PP	499.15^{bc}	904.01^{b}	5.32^{b}	6.67^{ab}	6.74^{bc}	8.84^{a}
	± 7.45	± 9.26	± 0.05	± 0.05	± 0.06	± 0.08
LL x WW	492.17^{bc}	914.00^{ab}	5.18^{cd}	6.82^{a}	6.56^{cde}	8.90^{a}
	± 8.30	± 9.10	± 0.05	± 0.06	± 0.08	± 0.09

PP x WW	468.04^{de} ± 8.23	865.84^{c} ± 9.83	5.13^{d} ± 0.06	6.60^{bc} ± 0.07	6.37^{e} ± 0.08	8.50^{c} ± 0.09
PP x LL	478.68^{cd} ± 8.52	896.54^{b} ± 11.44	5.10^{d} ± 0.06	6.40^{d} ± 0.09	6.45^{de} ± 0.09	8.66^{abc} ± 0.12
WW x LL	522.16^{a} ± 6.83	930.77^{a} ± 7.30	5.27^{bc} ± 0.06	6.82^{a} ± 0.06	6.61^{cd} ± 0.08	8.87^{a} ± 0.08
WW x PP	502.83^{bc} ± 6.36	898.89^{b} ± 7.81	5.16^{cd} ± 0.06	6.64^{b} ± 0.06	6.46^{de} ± 0.07	8.54^{bc} ± 0.09

Note: LL: Lavender, PP: Pearl, WW: White
Figures bearing similar superscript do not differ significantly (P<0.05) with each other

Table 5.20 : Mean heterosis in body weight and confirmation traits at different weeks of age in all possible crossbred groups under a full di-allele mating

Genetic groups (Sire x Dam)	Body eight (g) at		Shank length (cm) at		Keel length (cm) at	
	8th wk	12th wk	8th wk	12th wk	8th wk	12th wk
LL x PP	2.53	9.24	-4.32	2.34	-4.33	1.43
LL x WW	-5.81	10.96	-6.50	2.86	-7.93	1.48
PP x WW	-1.47	4.49	-7.23	1.30	-9.00	-2.02
PP x LL	-1.68	8.34	-8.27	-1.76	-8.45	-0.63
WW x LL	-0.07	13.00	-4.87	2.86	-7.23	1.14
WW x PP	5.85	8.48	-6.69	1.92	-7.71	-1.56

The highly significant (P< 0.01) specific combining ability estimates for body weight at 12 wk reflect the importance of non-additive gene effects (Kumar et al., 1997). Existence of significant reciprocal effects (RE) for 12 wk body weight further suggested sex-linked and maternal gene effects for this trait. Observation of negative reciprocal effect in case of White x

Lavender cross and maximum heterosis and highest specific combining ability (SCA) effect for Lavender x White crosses indicated the superiority of Lavender as male and White as female parents (Table 3.10). Another study of 'Guncari' germplasm also reported a higher degree of heterosis (7.37%) for the F1 crosses of Lavender and Pearl as compared to Pearl x Lavender crosses; which further support the use of Lavender as male parent.

Table 5.21 : General Combining Ability, specific Combining Ability and reciprocal effects estimated from a complete di-allele mating

Genetic groups	Body eight (g) at		Shank length (cm) at		Keel length (cm) at	
(Sire x Dam)	8th wk	12th wk	8th wk	12th wk	8th wk	12th wk
Over all means	497.60 ± 2.60	885.99 ± 3.31	5.32 ± 0.02	6.66 ± 0.02	6.79 ± 0.02	8.73 ± 0.03
General Combining Ability						
LL x LL	15.99^{a**}	5.10^{a}	0.023^{a}	0.056^{a**}	0.077^{a**}	0.097^{a**}
PP x PP	-22.94^{**}	-4.95^{a}	-0.008^{a}	-0.090^{b**}	-0.062^{b**}	-0.091^{b**}
WW x WW	6.94^{b**}	-0.15^{a}	-0.015^{a}	0.034^{a*}	-0.015^{b}	-0.007^{b}
Specific Combining Ability						
LL x PP	1.70^{a*}	23.46^{b**}	-0.115^{a**}	0.062^{a*}	-0.128^{a**}	0.022^{a}
LL x WW	-9.93^{b**}	40.70^{a**}	-0.095^{a**}	0.075^{a**}	-0.185^{a**}	0.078^{a}
PP x WW	7.27^{a*}	10.81^{b*}	-0.138^{a**}	0.017^{a}	-0.210^{a**}	-0.103^{b*}
Reciprocal effects						
PP x LL	10.23^{a*}	3.74^{ab}	0.111^{a**}	-0.015^{a}	0.145^{a**}	0.094^{a}
WW x LL	-14.99^{b**}	-8.39^{b}	-0.044^{b}	0.002^{a}	-0.028^{b}	0.016^{a}
WW x PP	-17.39^{b**}	-16.53^{a*}	-0.015^{b}	-0.017^{a}	-0.049^{b}	-0.024^{a}

Figures bearing similar superscript do not differ significantly ($P<0.05$) with each other

*: significant estimate ($P < 0.05$), **: significant estimate ($P < 0.01$)

❒❒❒

Chapter **6**

Immunogenetics

Immunity and Immune system

Immunity can be broadly classified as Innate and adaptive. The innate immunity is the first line of defense against invading pathogen and is of non-specific type, triggered by danger signals. The cells involved are leucocytes, natural killer cell and the mediator proteins are complement proteins, acute phase proteins, adhesion proteins, radicals, oxides, lysozymes, surfactants, lectins etc. The adaptive immunity occurs as second line of defense and is of specific types. The cells involved are antigen presenting cells, B cells and T cells. The mediator proteins are major histocompatability complex

(MHC), T cell receptors, B cell receptors, antibodies, cytokines etc. The variation in immune response between populations/ individuals is linked to the structural and functional diversity of the mediator proteins. These proteins are encoded by various genes such as Major Histocompatability Complex (MHC), T cell Receptors, Cytokines etc.

Genes Influencing Disease Resistance

Major Histocompatability Complex (MHC)

The MHC in chicken comprises of most polymorphic three closely linked genetic loci. These MHC genes determine the enconding of proteins, found on the plasmalemma of all body cells; proteins specific to the B-cells, T-cells and certain phagocytes; and also the complement system. This multi-allelic locus also plays important role in determination of immune response functions and disease resistance etc. B-blood group system of chicken is an important component of the major histocompatibility complex (MHC).

Haemagglutination tests of guinea fowl red cells with 10 chicken B-blood group reagents obtained from Iowa State University, Ames, Iowa revealed high incidence of positive reactions eg- B2-1.0, B6-0.6, B13-1.0, B19-1.0, BE-0.5, BF-0.6, Bj-0.7, Bx-1.0. These results suggest wide spread presence of antigenic specificities similar/corresponding to B blood groups of chicken.

Similar observations were made during another blood group Investigation conducted in collaboration with The Institute of Basic Animal Sciences, Humboldt University, Berlin. Haemagglutination tests of guinea fowl red-cells (n-12) with specific antisera for identification of chicken B-F (Class-1) and B-G (Class IV) heliotypes (allelic forms) viz. F2, F4, F12, F14, F15, F19, F21 and G12, G19, G21 respectively revealed 100% incidence of similar/corresponding antigenic specificities. Few antisera (F4, F12, F13, F14, G19, G21) showed distinctly higher degree of reactivity (++) than the remaining. These preliminary characterizations of guinea fowl red cells with chicken specific MHC-antisera suggested existence of little individual variations. In view of the fact that such monospecific antisera show different pattern of reactions when used for testing of, populations other than the reference populations, no precise inferences could be drawn on the basis of presently observed multiple reactivity (cross reactivity) but these results suggest existence of possible antigenic configurational relationships. Present protocol together with graft-versus-host (GVH) pock assay might prove useful first step for production of monospecific antisera for identification of guinea fowl red-cell specificities.

Disease Resistance

General Immunocompetence

Information on general or specific disease resistance potentials is the most desirable approach for disease control. Demands are strong for genetic stocks with greater disease resistance and higher responses to vaccines. Indigenous guinea fowl germplasm has a distinct reputation for natural disease resistance potentials. Natural immunity involves interactions of T-cell mediated immunity, non cellular humoral immunity and phagocytosis. Attempts were made to study the immune status parameters representing all the three immunity facts.

Existence of wide ranging individual variations were observed for serum Ig-G level, haemolytic and bactericidal complement levels, serum lysozyme level and the status of phagocytic activity in indigenous guinea fowl germplasm (Saxena, 1993). Mean values, varietal and sex differences and age related trends are presented in Table 6.1. Attempts to study genetic and non-genetic factors affecting these traits revealed significant differences due to age. Immune response to nonspecific multideterminant complex antigens like sheep erythrocytes (SRBCs) or simple nonspecific lymphocytic stimulants such as phytohaemagglutinin-P (PHA-P) and concavalin-A (Con-A) provide good indication of cellular immunocompetence. Mean values for non-specific immunity components of serum and in vivo response to Con-A and PHA-P measured as wing index (WI) and immune response titre to SRBCs (sheep red blood cells 1 ml I/v) were comparable or higher than that obtained for indigenous fowl (Kadaknath) and commercial broilers (Saxena, 1993).

In another study, Phagocytic index revealed significant differences between varieties. Lavender showed highest phagocytic index (0.071 ±0.005) followed by Pearl (0.061 ±0.004) and White (0.051 ±0.005). Similarly, response to PHA-P was highest in Pearl, followed by White, while Lavender variety showed minimum response to PHA-P. However, antibody response to SRBC as well as complement level in serum did not differed significantly between varieties. For all these parameters, no significant difference was found between the rapid feathering and slow feathering birds. Similarly the variety X feathering type interaction was also non-significant (Table 6.2).

Table 6.1 : Mean estimates of different measures of general immune competence in guinea fowl

Immune traits	Verities			Sex		Overall estimate
	White	Lavender	Pearl	Male	Female	
A. Humoral Immunity components (serum):						
Immunoglobulin level (mg/ml serum	12.4±0.3	12.3±0.2	11.7±0.2	12.2±0.1	12.2±0.1	12.2±0.1
Component activity level (log 10 (n+1)						
Haemolytic comp.	1.43±0.03	1.47±0.03	1.47±0.03	1.47±0.02	1.42±0.04	1.43±0.02
Bactericidal comp.	1.44±0.03	1.45±0.03	1.21±0.26	1.24±0.28	1.41±0.02	1.47±0.02
Lysozyme level	1.18±0.05	1.19±0.05	1.23±0.05	1.11±0.04	1.24±0.4	1.18±0.03
Cellular immune response to antigens:						
Response to Con - A	1.35±0.03	1.38±0.03	1.40±0.03	1.54±0.02	1.22±0.02	1.37±0.02
Response to PHA - P	0.63±0.03	0.58±0.05	0.65±0.04	0.65±0.04	0.56±0.03	0.61±0.03
Response to Sheep RBCs.	1.71±0.07	1.44±0.07	1.45±0.07	1.49±0.57	1.57±0.05	1.53±0.014
Phagocytic index	0.19±0.01	0.19±0.01	0.19±0.01	0.18±0.01	0.19±0.01	0.19±0.01

Table 6.2 : Mean ± SE for various immuno-competence traits in guinea fowl

No. of	Complement level in serum	Response to SRBC	Response to PHA-P	Phagocytic Index
Overall	1.63 ±0.010	1.68 ±0.016	0.64 ±0.001	.061 ±0.002
Varieties				
Lavender	1.65 ±0.018	1.70 ±0.028	0.59 ±0.002	.071 ±0.005
Pearl	1.65 ±0.018	1.65 ±0.027	0.68 ±0.002	.061 ±0.004
White	1.60 ±0.019	1.70 0.028	0.66 ±0.002	.051 ±0.005
Feathering rate				
RF	1.64 ±0.013	1.66 ±0.020	0.65 ±0.001	.062 ±0.003
SF	1.62 ±0.017	1.70 ±0.025	0.64 ±0.002	.060 ±0.004

Variety X Feathering rate				
Lavender RF	1.67 ±0.022	1.65 ±0.034	0.60 ±0.003	.079 ±0.006
Lavender SF	1.62 ±0.030	1.75 ±0.045	0.58 ±0.004	.063 ±0.008
Pearl RF	1.67 ±0.023	1.61 ±0.034	0.68 ±0.003	.056 ±0.006
Pearl SF	1.62 ±0.028	1.68 ±0.042	0.69 ±0.003	.067 ±0.007
White RF	1.58 ±0.024	1.73 ±0.037	0.68 ±0.003	.053 ±0.006
White SF	1.62 ±0.029	1.68 ±0.044	0.64 ±0.003	.050 ±0.008

Note: RF: Rapid feathering, SF: Slow Feathering

The antibody response to SRBC, estimated in terms of antibody HA titer showed a specific trend in post immunization period (Sharma 2007). Among the different age groups at all dpi, the HA titre was maximum at 11 wk of age, however they were non-significantly different with the HA titers at 9 wk of age, but significantly different with the HA titter at 13 wks of age (Fig 6.1). The HA titre at 6th weeks of age were significantly lower than other age groups at all days post immunization. At 5 days post immunization, the differences among different age groups were not much pronounced as the HA titre at 9 wk, 11 wk and 13 wk were non significantly different with each other. The HA titre at 6th week was though significantly lower than the titers at 11th wk and 13th wk, but not with titre at 9th wk of age. For persistency of the titre, at all the weeks of age, maximum titre was observed at 8 dpi, which was then declined

significantly at 12 dpi and further declined significantly at 15 dpi (Fig 6.1). However at 6th wk of age, maximum titre was attained at earlier period i.e. 5 dpi and persisted at same level at 8 dpi and then dropped significantly at 12 and 15 dpi. These results suggest that optimum age for estimating response to SRBC is between 9 – 11 weeks of age and the antibody titre reaches to maximum peak at 8 days post immunization.

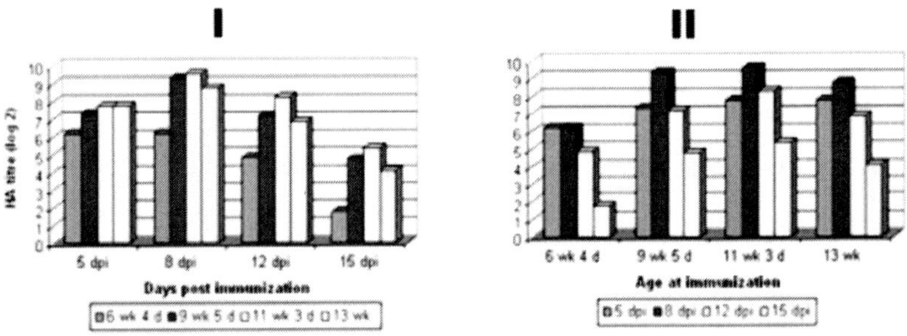

Fig. 6.1 : I. Days post immunization wise mean HA titre at different ages at immunization. II. Age at immunization wise mean HA titre at different days post immunization

Existence of significant sire effect and moderate heritability estimates indicate considerable role of additive gene components (Table 6.3). Inheritance studies among progeny from mating between parents with known high or low phenotypes further suggest existence of dominant major gene(s) influences also. Present immune-competence results in guinea fowl indicate distinct similarity with genetic determination of these traits in chicken (Saxena, 1993; Singh et al., 1996).

Table 6.3 : Heritability estimates for immune-competence

Immune traits	Sire families	K value	Heritability level
Immunoglobulin (Ig-G) level	28	8.1	0.18±0.14
Haemolytic complement level	28	6.2	0.04±0.11
Bactericidal complement level	28	5.7	0.07±0.11
Lysozyme level	28	7.1	0.36±0.17
Response to SRBCs.	28	7.2	0.35±0.17
Response to Con - A	28	10.9	0.27±0.16
Response to PHA - P	28	6.5	0.03±0.20
Phagocytic index:	28	10.9	0.17±0.13

Associations between immunological traits are important when breeding for disease resistance is aimed. Correlations between cellular and humoral immunity traits were mostly if low order, but high genetic correlations were obtained for complement level (haemolytic and bactericidal) with lysozyme level and immune response to SRBCs; and also between phagocytic index and immune response to Con-A. These observations are in good agreement with earlier report for chicken but further studies are desired in view of relatively high standard errors observed in these investigations.

Immunocompetence & survivability: Immuno-logically superior birds show relative superior survivability; higher level of immune-competence lead to lower mortality. The correlations of various traits with sire wise mortality showed high negative values which ranged from -0.74 to 0.07 (Saxena, 1993). The mortality percentage among sire progeny groups were low where sire showed high levels of immune-competence status and vice versa (Table 6.4).

Table 6.4 : Immunity traits and average mortality among progeny of sires ranked high/medium/low for mmuno-competence traits

Immune competence traits	Average mortality %			Correlation
	High	Medium	Low	
Response to SRBCs.	1.2	4.6	10.5	-0.74
Serum Ig-G level	3.0	5.3	6.4	0.07
Haemolytic complement	4.6	4.5	10.5	0.01
Bactericidal complement	4.5	5.2	8.0	0.01
Serum Lysozyme level	1.9	4.5	6.2	-0.04
Phagocytic index	1.6	7.4	10.6	-0.05
Wing Index	1.5	6.2	8.0	-0.25
Av. Mortality (%)	2.6	5.4	8/6	

Investigations with three weight free selection indices constructed on humoral immunity traits i.e. Optima-HI; Optima-CMI for cell mediated immunity traits and IR-Optima based on all the six traits (Saxena, 1993)

showed that mortality among progeny of the sires ranked on the basis of above indices were -0.31, -0.36 and -0.37 for Optima-HI, Optima-CMI and IR-Optima respectively (Table 6.5).

Table 6.5 : Immuno-competence index associations with survivability

Characters	Targeted Index values		
	Optima-HI (17.93)	Optima-CMI (12.97)	IR-Optima (26.95)
No. of selected sire families	31	34	13
Mortality in sire progeny (%)	1.5	1.6	1.2
Improvement over total mortality in flock (%)	72	71	78
RIM	-0.31	-0.36	-0.37

Egg components and antimicrobial defenses: Each egg is a potential keet; therefore microbial load of egg contents has direct influence on the embryonic viability. Developing embryos possess a series of non-specific defense mechanisms to ensure a contaminant free environment inside the egg. These include i. the physical barriers imposed by shell and related structures which impede the microbial entries, and ii. Chemical defense mechanisms extended by biochemical components of egg white which restrict microbial colonization and their subsequent rapid growth. It is well accepted that freshly laid egg is sterile in 95% of the cases. The contamination starts subsequently after the egg comes in contact with external environment; and it is proportional to the environmental pollution. Present investigations showed that the above mentioned antimicrobial defenses were relatively better developed in case of guinea fowl. Assessment of mean total aerobic microbial load on egg shell surface (1.96 ± 0.03 log10 CFU/cm^2) and internal contents (1.25 ± 0.01 log10 CFU/gm) revealed statistically significant variations between individual eggs from same hen and between eggs from different hens (Sajjnar, 1994). Microbial load of internal contents represent nearly 24% of the total shell load (Table 6.6) and both are also correlated significantly (r-0.06; P< 0.05) (Anand et al., 1993).

It was further observed that physical quality traits and biochemical components of egg associated with non-specific anti-microbial defenses also revealed negative correlations with microbial load of egg contents (assessed as percentage of shell loads) e.g. lysozyme (r-0.18, h^2 0.77 ± 0.16); conalbumin (r-0.18, h^2 0.25 ± 0.22); ovalbumin (r-0.22, h^2 0.20 ± 0.24); albumen index (r-0.06, h^2 0.34 ± 0.12); shell thickness (r-0.06, h^2 0.49 ± 0.14); shell porosity (r-0.08, h^2 0.52 ± 0.14) and shell membrane thickness (r-0.01, h^2 0.56 ± 0.14). Gene determined ovoalbumen phenotype variations (Ov-AA, Ov-AB, Ov-BB types) revealed no significant influence on the microbial load of the egg contents. These results emphasize the functional importance of the non-specific antimicrobial barriers in restricting the microbial entries and also as effective impediment to their rapid multiplication. The moderate heritability values obtained for these traits indicate the improvement possibilities through routine breeding approaches (Sajjnar, 1994).

Specific Disease Resistance

Specific disease resistance is the ability to overcome or to tolerate a specific infection with little or no adverse effects on health status. Guinea fowl has a reputation of resistance to many common poultry diseases but precise knowledge of genetic system influences and the way in which they govern the host's responses is very limited. Present preliminary investigations in guinea fowl indicated relatively better developed 'thresholds' of specific responses to several avian pathogens.

Table 6.6 : Mean microbial loads observed among the groups identified high or low for antimicrobial defense traits in guinea fowl eggs

Traits	Herita-bility (h^2 S+D)	Cut off value for High / Low group	Microbial Load		Correlations	
			Shell surface (log CFU/cm^2)	Egg white (log CFU/gm)	Microb. load of content	Microb. load contents (% shell load)
I. Physical defense mechanism:						
Shell thickness (mm)	0.09± 0.14	High > 0.5	1.7±0.07	1.2±0.07	-0.03	-0.06
		Low < 0.3	2.1±0.06	1.3±0.06		
Shell porosity (pores/cm^2)	0.52± 0.14	High > 55.0	1.8±0.01	1.1±0.03	-0.06	-0.08
		Low < 35.0	1.6±0.02	1.2±0.03		
Shell memb. thick. (mm)	0.56± 0.14	High > 0.04	1.8±0.14	1.1±0.03	-0.05	-0.08
		Low < 0.03	1.9±0.09	1.2±0.05		
Haugh unit	0.31± 0.12	High > 85.0	1.9±0.62	1.2±0.38	-0.05	-0.08
		Low < 70.0	1.6±0.60	1.2±0.47		
II. Chemical defense mechanism:						
Ovalbumin level (%)	0.20± 0.24	High > 70.0	1.8±0.05	1.2±0.06	-0.07	-0.22
		Low < 60.0	1.9±0.08			
Ovoglobulin+Ovo mucoid (%)	0.13± 0.20	High > 16.0	1.9±0.08	1.3±0.06	-0.09	-0.08
		Low < 11.0	1.9±0.09	1.3±0.04		
Conalbumin level (%)	0.25± 0.22	High > 25.0	1.9±0.12	1.2±0.02	-0.16	-0.19
		Low < 16.0	1.8±0.09	1.3±0.06		
Lysozyme level (mg/ml)	0.77± 0.16	High > 2.5	1.9±0.08	1.3±0.06	-0.13	-0.18
		Low < 1.5	1.9±0.08	1.3±0.06		

Resistance to Leucosis Virus Infection: Genetic resistance to avian leucosis viruses (ALV) is a complex phenomenon. In case of domestic fowl resistance and susceptibility to ALV infections is under the control of singe gene(s) with genotypes which are specific for each group of avian leucosis virus. Using chorioallantoic membrane test (CAM- test) and liver tumor assay approaches, resistance to subgroup-A Rous sarcoma virus (RSV-A) was assessed in guinea fowl, White leghorn, numigal (Ch x GF hybrid) and a reference germplasm viz. White leghorn-SPF, ALC-negative, with 100% susceptibility to RSV-A (Venkateshwara Hatcheries, Pune). Studies of 464 guinea fowl CAMs inoculated with RSV-A showed a range of 0 to few pock marks (59%). Average pock count values of 17.7 ± 6.3, 173.4 ± 20.4 68.9 ± 8.3 and ∝ (infinite) respectively for the above four genetic groups. Population distribution for CAM- test results in guinea fowl eggs was distinctly bimodal. Sire-effects were highly significant but varietal differences and replicate effects were not significant. CAM- test results showed that WLH (SPF) and WLH (CARI) were the most susceptible genetic groups to RSV-A infections and guinea fowl were almost resistant; while numigal showed an intermediate susceptibility status (Table 6.7).

RSV-A inoculated eggs showed significant reduction in hatchability: 41%, 46% respectively in guinea fowl and WLH; and the distinctly low hatchability (15%) of chicken & guinea fowl was further reduced by 67%. Observed mortality among 2 wk old keets and chicks hatched from RSV-A inoculated eggs was 4.8% and 100% respectively; obviously the reaction of RSV-A was very mild among surviving keet. Conversely associated phenotypes (CAPs) i.e. CAM (+) and LT (-) were 76%, while all WLH (SPF) chicks exhibited CAM (+) and LT (+) phenotype. Necropsy results of keets killed at 4 and 8 wk age showed little incidence of liver tumors; histopathological investigations of visceral organs also revealed no incidence of pathological lesions. On other hand the post mortem results for WLH (SPF) chicks showed profuse tumor growths in liver and similar lesions in all visceral organs. Numigal keets also showed relatively high death incidence within 7-12 days of post hatching, liver tumors were also profuse but comparatively much less than the WLH (SPF) chicks. Relative susceptibility estimates: 0.09%, 0.39% and 0.61% observed respectively for guinea fowl, numigal and Desi fowl in comparison to WLH (CARI) suggest existence of high resistance to the RSV infections in guinea fowl (Saxena, 1993). Another study reported six times less susceptibility for guinea fowl stock as compared to WLH; average pock counts reported for guinea fowl, Aseel and Kadaknath were : 37.1, 46.5 and 96.8 respectively. In guinea fowl all four phenotypes were identified. The percentage of conversely associated phenotypes were 69.3% while in White leghorn the CAM (+) and LT (+) phenotype was 46.2% (Rout, 1990).

Table 6.7 : Estimation of resistance to subgroup-A Rous Sarcoma virus

	Average pock count	Range	Relative susceptibility	Gene freq. (q^{ar})
A. CAM test results:				
i. Guinea fowl				
Lavender	17.7±4.1	0 to 105	-	-
Pearl	15.1±9.2	0 to 102	-	-
White	21.6±3.6	0 to 120	-	-
Overall	17.7±6.3	0 to 120	0.09	0.77
ii. White Leghorn (CARI)	173.4±20.3	80 to x	1.00	0.00
iii. White Leghorn (SPF-ALC-ve)	Infinite	-	1.00	0.00
iv. Numigal (Ch x GF)	68.9±8.3	0 to > 200	0.39	0.46

B. Liver tumor assay results:

	Hatchability%		Percent non-reactors	Tumor incidence (%)	Mortality percent (up to 6 wk)
	Control	Exptl. group			
i. Guinea fowl	70	41	35.0	00.0	4.8
ii. White Leghorn (CARI)	80	46	00.0	100.0	100.0
iii. Numigal (Ch x GF)	18	6	10.0	80.0	90.0
iv. White Leghorn (SPF-ALC-ve)	80	43	00.0	100.0	100.0

The Leucosis 'Shedder' Status: Information regarding the incidence of 'shedders' of group specific leucosis antigen (GSA) in egg albumen is an important approach for identification of congenital transmission of avian leucosis sarcoma viruses (ALSV) infection. Routine monitoring of diversified poultry germplasm is normally done by detection of group specific antigen (GSA) by complement fixation for avian leucosis (COFAL) test or through the use of ALS virus antigen specific enzyme-linked immunosorbent assay

(ELISA) employing egg white. Investigations with several poultry species (Panisup et al., 1990) showed that all guinea fowl samples were negative for the group specific leucosis antigen and therefore free from infection (Table 6.8). This significant observation further supports the genetic resistance of guinea fowl to ALS virus infections.

Table 6.8 : Monitoring of avian leucosis- Sarcoma group specific viral antigen (AL-Sv gs AG) in the egg white

Genetic groups	COFAL +ve (%)	COFAL -ve (%)
Guinea fowl (Guncari)	nil	100.0
Desi fowl	35.2	64.8
White leghorn	62.2	37.8
Rhode Island red	57.3	42.7
Quail	Nil	100.0
Duck	nil	100.0

In chicken the susceptibility to RSV–A is related to presence of appropriate virus receptors on the host cell surface under single gene control where susceptibility gene (as) is partially dominant over the resistance determining gene (ar). In guinea fowl and numigal, the gene frequency of ar allele is 0.77 and 0.36 respectively. Observation of moderate heritability estimate (0.41± 0.01) for incidence of pock marks in guinea fowl and low susceptibility for numigal (mid way between the two parent species) possible indicate a homologous location for the focus determining resistance in the two species.

Resistance to Marek's Disease (MD): This lymphoproliferative disease caused by herpes virus is extremely contagious and spreads horizontally. Marek's disease has been responsible for major economic losses in chicken and is also known to affect guinea fowl. An assay of pathogen specific antibodies in blood provides a good method to determine whether a flock has previously encountered the pathogens and has mounted an immune response. Preliminary studies in guinea fowl indicated higher "species specific threshold" to Marek's disease virus infection also. Serological studies (ELISA test and virus neutralization test) conducted with guinea fowl serum from normal individual revealed complete absence of corresponding antibody. These observations in un-vaccinated guinea fowl flock which is being maintained among the routinely vaccinated chicken certainly has some relevance to speculate better developed resistance of guinea fowl to the Marek's disease virus infection.

Of particular importance is the observation regarding the absence of ev-21 locus in case of guinea fowl. The ev-21 gene (closely linked with slow feathering allele in case of domestic fowl) is known to influence response to ALV infections and perhaps increase the viraemia and shedder status.

Studies in domestic fowl show that the genetic constitution of host has strong influences on response to MDV infections. Breeders have successfully selected stocks with reduced susceptibility to MDV. This gene determined reduced susceptibility is not resistance to infection but it is resistance to the development of disease after infection. It may be either due to influence of major histocompatibility complex alleles which provide better immune response or it might be through susceptibility of T-cells to transformation.

Resistance to Newcastle Disease : Ranikhet disease (RD) or Newcastle disease (ND), is a highly devastating disease responsible for extensive mortality among poultry birds. Breed or genetic stock of domestic fowl has little influence on the susceptibility to ND virus, but duck and geese however show few or no clinical signs even with strains highly lethal for chicken. Investigations showed that guinea fowl are relatively less susceptible. Although reared along with highly susceptible layer and broiler stocks; un-vaccinated guinea fowl revealed no Newcastle disease out breaks. The pathogenicity tests with different ND virus isolates provided useful information regarding the species specific differences in susceptibility.

A detailed knowledge of the pathogen and its interactions with susceptible or resistant host is the first desirable pre-requisite for identification of disease resistance potentials. Relatively better resistance of guinea fowl was observed during two different controlled experimental infection studies with New castle disease virus in guinea fowl and chicken. Experimental infection with a velogenic - viscerotropic New castle disease virus isolate from guinea fowl (viz. GNDV AD-18/92 which showed 100 percent antigenic relationship with chicken virus CNDV AD-75 during cross haemagglutination inhibition test) indicated relatively low susceptibility for guinea fowl as compared to chicken. Oronasal inoculations of this virus in chickens produced disease symptoms marked by white diarrhoea, tremors of legs and wings followed by paralysis, and mortality was around 60%. The presence of virus in intestine and cloacal contents indicated excretion of virus through feces. Histo-pathological examinations revealed non-purulent encephalitis; necrosis and depletion on of lymphoid tissue in spleen, Bursa of Fabricius, caecal tonsilitis, mild haemorrhages at the tip of the glands of proventriculus, hyperplasia of bronchiolar epithelium and mild interlobular oedema in lung. This virus also produced disease in guinea fowls but all symptoms were comparatively mild and nervous symptoms were moderate. Little specific gross changes were observed except mild haemorrhages seen at tip of the gland in proventriculus and caecal tonsils in few birds. Histopathological lesions were also much less severe which consisted of mild haemorrhages, depletion of lymphoid cells and necrosis of lymphoid tissues in bursa of Fabrigius and other glands. Some mild changes were also observed in lung, trachea and cerebellum. No changes were identified in spleen, liver and kidneys. As compared to chickens the mortality was also significantly less (30%) (Kinderle, 1994).

In another detailed study, investigated comparative pathogenicity of three different ND virus isolates from chicken (CNDV), guinea fowl

(GNDV) and pigeon (PNDV) in guinea fowl (Misra, 1997). Results showed only mild clinical symptoms in guinea fowl as compared to chicken. Mortality rate was high (52%) in case of CNDV infected group, whereas most of the birds infected with GNDV and PNDV recovered after showing early clinical symptoms; only 8% mortality was observed (Table 6.9). All the isolates produced good level of antibody response in guinea fowl.

Table 6.9 : Morbidity and mortality pattern following incubation with three different N. D. virus isolates (dose oronsal 10^6 EID_{50}/0.1/ml isolates)

Species/ State after inoculation	Days post infection 4	5	6	7	8	9	10	11	12	13	19	20	Reco-very DPI	Mort-ality %
CNDV-Inoculations														
Keets (4wk)														
Sick	-	2	3	11	6	4	1	1	1	1	-	-	13	52
Paralyze	-	-	2	4	9	7	10	5	1	-	-	-		
Dead	-	1	-	1	-	4	-	5	1	1	-	-		
Chickens (3wk)														
Sick	2	3	18	6	7	6	2	-	-	-	-	-	10	56
Paralyze	-	-	3	8	-	-	-	-	-	-	-	-		
Dead	-	1	-	7	6	1	2	-	-	-	-	-		
GNDV-Inoculations														
Keets (4wk)														
Sick	-	1	-	3	3	-	-	-	-	-	-	-	8	8
Paralyze	-	-	6	3	-	-	-	-	-	-	-	-		
Dead	-	-	-	2	-	-	-	-	-	-	-	-		
Chickens (3wk)														
Sick	3	4	5	5	5	6	6	3	7	4	-	-	14	56
Paralyze	-	-	1	1	1	-	-	3	-	-	-	-		
Dead	-	1	2	-	-	1	1	3	5	4	-	-		

PNDV-Inoculations														
Keets (4wk)														
Sick	-	-	-	-	-	-	-	-	-	-	-	-	13	8
Paralyze	-	-	1	-	-	-	-	-	-	-	-	-		
Dead	-	-	-	1	-	-	-	-	-	1	-	-		
Chickens (3wk)														
Sick	-	-	2	-	-	-	-	-	-	-	1	-	24	6
Paralyze	-	-	-	-	-	-	-	-	-	-	-	-		
Dead	-	-	-	1	-	-	-	-	-	-	-	1		

The antibody titre against RD virus, determined as total haemagglutination (HA) titre, 2-ME sensitive antibody (IgM) and 2-ME resistant antibody (IgG) were studied. While, effect of sex and interaction between sex and variety found revealed significant for total HA titre and 2 ME sensitive titre, feathering rate influenced 2-ME resistant antibody (IgG) significantly (Table 6.10). Therefore, the total HA titers were higher in males and the differences between sexes were more prominent in Lavender variety. The rapid feathering birds showed higher initial IgG titre in comparison to the slow feathered birds.

Resistance to Tick Infestations: Apparently common and widely prevalent *Argus persicus* is known to parasitize a variety of birds. This tick is a natural vector of the spirochaete *Borrelia anserina* and *Aegioptionella pullorum*. Infestations by larval and adult stages cause paralysis in chicks. Experimental infections with

Table 6.10 : Effect of variety, rate of feathering and their interactions on antibody responses against RD virus.

	Before inoculation			10 d post inoculation		
	Total Ig	IgG	IgM	Total Ig	IgG	IgM
Overall	2.18±0.09	1.25±0.05	0.92±0.09	2.90±0.08	1.31±0.05	1.59±0.09
Variety						
Leaveder	1.98±0.15	1.25±0.08	0.73±0.16	2.98±0.14	1.38±0.09	1.59±0.16
Pearl	2.20±0.16	1.22±0.08	0.97±0.16	2.87±0.14	1.27±0.09	1.59±0.16
White	2.37±0.14	1.30±0.08	1.07±0.15	2.90±0.13	1.29±0.09	1.60±0.15
Sex						
Male	2.35±0.12	1.24±0.06	1.10±0.12	2.79±0.11	1.27±0.07	1.52±0.13
Female	2.02±0.11	1.27±0.06	0.75±0.11	3.04±0.10	1.36±0.07	1.67±0.12
Feathering rate						
RF	2.13±0.15	1.34±0.08	0.78±0.15	2.84±0.14	1.34±0.09	1.50±0.15
SF	2.24±0.09	1.17±0.05	1.06±0.09	2.99±0.08	1.29±0.05	1.69±0.10
Variety x Sex						
L.M	2.44±0.20	1.32±0.11	1.11±0.21	2.99±0.19	1.34±0.12	1.64±0.22
L.F	1.52±0.21	1.17±0.11	0.35±0.21	2.97±0.20	1.42±0.13	1.54±0.22
Pearl male	2.17±0.25	1.16±0.13	1.02±0.25	2.48±0.23	1.11±0.15	1.37±0.26
Pearl female	2.23±0.17	1.28±0.09	0.92±0.17	3.25±0.15	1.44±0.10	1.81±0.18
White male	2.42±0.19	1.25±0.10	1.16±0.19	2.90±0.18	1.34±0.12	1.55±0.21
White female	2.32±0.21	1.34±0.11	0.97±0.21	2.90±0.19	1.24±0.13	1.65±0.22
Variety x Feathering rate						
Lavender RF	1.83±0.27	1.40±0.15	0.43±0.28	3.08±0.25	1.58±0.17	1.49±0.29
Lavender SF	2.13±0.16	1.09±0.09	1.03±0.17	2.87±0.15	1.17±0.10	1.70±0.17
Pearl	2.29±0.26	1.28±0.14	1.01±0.27	2.77±0.25	1.24±0.16	1.53±0.28
Pearl	2.10±0.16	1.16±0.09	0.92±0.16	2.96±0.149	1.31±0.10	1.65±0.17
White	2.25±0.24	1.34±0.13	0.91±0.25	2.66±0.226	1.18±0.15	1.47±0.25
White	2.50±0.17	1.26±0.09	1.23±0.17	3.13±0.159	1.40±0.10	1.73±0.18

bacterial isolates from this tick have been found to cause serious disease conditions. Feeding behavior of *Argus persicus* adults and its developmental stages on domestic fowl (6-8.wk) and guinea fowl (8-10 wk) growers was studied by experimental exposure of the two groups (5 replicates) to known number of larvae, nymphs (1st and 2nd stages) and adults. Their subsequent recovery percentage showed statistically significant differences. In chicken hosts the larvae remain firmly attached to body especially under the wings and cause maximum damage by sucking blood for about a week. While in case of guinea fowl hosts these larvae did not attach readily and the number of larvae that was actually found feeding was also significantly less (fig 6.2). Although nymphs and adults showed similar feeding pattern on both the hosts but significant difference in larval feeding pattern underline the higher resistance of guinea fowl. (Srivastava and Singh, 1988, Srivastava, 1989).

In another investigation, analysis of data for three consecutive feeding trials with *A. persicus* larvae (10 day old) on guinea fowl growers (12 wk) revealed significant effects of number of feeding and sex on per cent larvae fed. Although highest values were observed for white birds (24.4± 3.2) but differences among varieties were not significant. The average time of attachment of larvae on the body of bird was 37.0± 3.3 hr (Figure 6.3). The larvae fed percentage were significantly less in case of males (20.3± 1.9) than females (24.8± 3.4). It was lowest during the third feeding (14.5± 1.9) compared to second (22.3± 3.5) and first (30.4± 3.2) feeding.

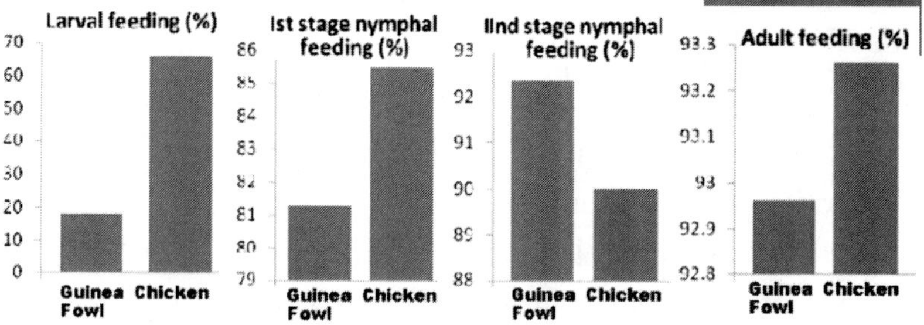

Fig. 6.2 : Percent larval, different stage of nymphs as well as adult feeding in guinea fowl and chicken

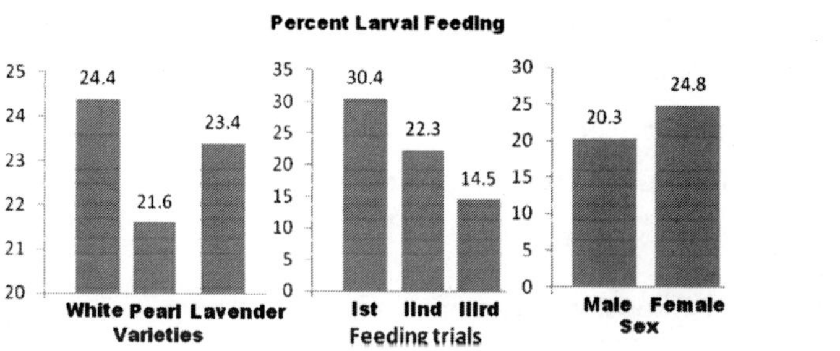

Fig. 6.3: Effect of variety, feeding trials and sexes on Percent larval feeding

The consistent fall in number of larvae fed during the consecutive feeding was observed in all individuals; who indicated development of acquired resistance in guinea fowl. The observed difference in larvae fed percentage between two sexes might be due to differences in immunity status and skin qualities in males and females (Saxena et al., 1996).

Resistance to Lice Infestations: In tropics, poultry lice (*Menonpon gallinae* and *Lipeurus tropicalis*) infestations are quite common. In chicken tangible economic losses in terms of weight gains, feed efficiency and egg production are usually attributed to intense body irritations caused during lice infestation.

A comparison of growth performance of 'Guncari' guinea fowl and Kadaknath chicken growers kept separately in two side by side pens heavily infested with common lice revealed significant reduction in body weight gains for the chicken host; while relatively little effect was detected for the guinea fowl growers (Table 6.11). Subject to further verifications these preliminary observations indicated relatively lower susceptibility of guinea fowl to the common lice species.

Table 6.11 : Resistance to common lice infestations

Genetic groups	Age in week	Body weight in g of birds reared in	
		Lice free pens	Lice Infested pen
Guinea fowl	4 wk	160±2.90^{a}	155±3.00^{a}
	8 wk	389.0±5.00^{a}	369.0±10.1^{a}
	12 wk	650±11.9^{a}	645.0±11.6^{a}
Kadak-nath	4 wk	170.3±5.10^{a}	150.3±10.1^{b}
	8 wk	405.8±18.0^{a}	376.8±19.9^{b}
	12 wk	750.1±20.0^{a}	685.9±24.0^{b}

Note : Figure bearing same superscripts do not differ significantly with each other.

❑❑❑

Chapter **7**

Molecular Genetics

Genome Size

Total amount of DNA contained within one copy of a genome is called genome size. It is expressed in terms of mass in expressed in picograms (10^{-12} of a gram) or less frequently in Daltons or more commonly as the total number of nucleotide base pairs (in bases or megabases, where 1 megabase is equal to millions of base pairs). The total amount of DNA in the haploid genome is called its C value and is expressed in pg. For inter-conversion, 1 picogram equals 978 megabases or 0.978 x 10^{9} bases pairs. In mammals, the size of the genome is more than 3 billion base pairs, while, avian genome is about one third of it i.e. ~ 1.2 billion bases pairs. The diploid cells i.e. somatic cells contain double of the DNA present in haploid cell. The genome sizes of some domesticated birds of economic importance are as follows.

Table 7.1 : Genome size in different poultry species

S No	Species	Common name	Number of chromosomes (2n)	C value	Genome size in base pairs
1	*Anas platyrhynchos*	Duck	80	1.44	1.41×10^9
2	*Coturnix japonica*	Japanese quail	78	1.41	1.38×10^9
3	*Gallus domesticus*	Domestic chicken	78	1.25	1.22×10^9
4	*Meleagris gallopavo*	Turkey	80	1.40	1.37×10^9
5	*Numida meleagris*	Guinea fowl	78	1.23	1.20×10^9
6	*Anser rossii*	Ross's goose	82	1.38	1.35×10^9
7	*Columba livia*	Rock pigeon	80	1.46	1.43×10^9
8	*Struthio camelus*	Ostrich	80	2.16	2.11×10^9
9	*Dromaius novaehollandiae*	Emu	80	1.63	1.59×10^9

Though, the genome size might seem to be a good indicator of the genetic content, or "complexity", but there is a remarkable lack of correspondence between genome size and organism complexity, specially in eukaryotes for example, the genome size of marbled lungfish

(*Protopterus aethiopicus*) is ~130 x 10^9 base pairs against the ~3 x 10^9 and ~1.2 x 10^9 base pairs in mammals and birds, respectively. Similarly, there is remarkable lack of correspondence between the number of protein-coding genes and organism complexity. While the human genome, for example, has about 20,000 to 25,000 protein-coding genes, *Trichomonas vaginalis,* a single-celled parasitic organism has approximately 60,000 protein-coding genes. It is felt that the numbers of protein-coding genes in eukaryotes are around 25,000 or so though the genome size may vary to the tune of 5-6 folds. In chicken (*Gallus gallus*), 20000-23000 protein coding genes are expected to be present and in guinea fowl, the number of genes is also expected to same.

Genome Organization

Genome organization refers to the sequential, not the structural organization of the genome. Mainly there are either coding sequences or non-coding sequences. While the coding sequences are the exons of the genes, the non-coding DNA may fall in the following classes

Introns: They are DNA sequences inserted between the exons and found in the ORF. They are spliced after the first level of transcription. Most introns are junk inserted within genes.

Pseudogenes: 'Dead', non-functional copies of genes present elsewhere in the genome, but no longer of any use.

Retropseudogenes: Like pseudogenes, but have been processed, i.e. lack introns. Produced by the action of reverse transcriptase (RT) on mRNA, and subsequent incorporation of the cDNA into the genome.

Transposons: Jumping genes, which splice themselves in and out of the genome (in DNA form) randomly, by the action of transposase.

Retrotransposons: Transcribed into an mRNA, which encodes an RT enzyme, which then copies the mRNA back to DNA and incorporates it into the genome.

In fact in humans only 1.5% of the entire genome length corresponds to coding DNA. This 1.5% codes for about 27,000 genes which in turn code for proteins that are responsible for all the cellular processes.

Organization of DNA sequences

In eukaryotic genomes, DNA sequences are represented at different levels of repetitions.

It may be single copy sequences, occurring once or a few times reoccurrence or highly repetitive DNA sequences, which are found from 100,000 to 1 million times in the genome. While the single copy sequences are mostly are functional genes encoding sequences, example of middle repetitive DNA sequences are rRNA and tRNA genes. The highly repetitive DNA sequences are found in regions of the chromosome such as heterochromatin, centromeres and telomeres and tend to be arranged as a tandem repeats.

If we denature the DNA, due to melting of H-bonds, the DNA become single stranded. Slow cooling of the denatured DNA allows the complementary sequences to reanneal. Plotting of the percent of the DNA that remains single stranded, expressed as a ratio of the concentration of single-stranded DNA (*C*) to the total concentration of the starting DNA (*Co*) against the X-axis, a log-scale of the product of the initial concentration of DNA (in moles/liter) multiplied by length of time the reaction proceeded (in seconds) and is called as "Cot", the obtained curve is called "Cot curve". One particular value that is useful is $Cot_{1/2}$, the *Cot* value where half of the DNA has reannealed. For the simple genome such as that of *E. coli* the curve is single and smooth. But for the genomes having all the three classes of sequences, "Cot" curve not single, but three distinct curves are seen and each curve represent a each class (Fig 7.1).

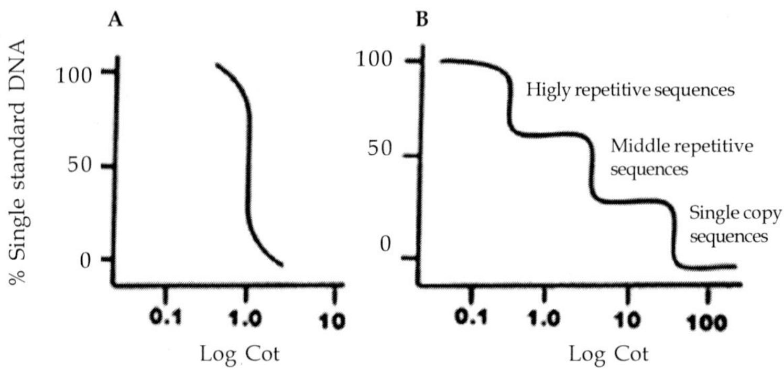

Fig. 7.1 : "Cot" curve of prokaryote (A) and eukaryote (B) organism

The order of reannealing depends upon the level of repetition, hence the highly reanneal first as there are high number of copies and such sequences are less complex. The second portion of the genome to reanneal is the middle repetitive DNA, and in last the genome portion having single copy sequences reanneal.

Avian genome organization

Like most bird species, the chicken has a relatively small genome of <1200 million base pairs (Mbp), or <39% of the size of the human genome. It has been suggested that an important factor in genome size reduction in birds has been that birds have lower levels of repetitive DNA than other vertebrates (Burt, 2002). Genomes of mammals and reptiles are estimated to consist of about 30–50% repeats, while those of birds have been estimated to consist of only 15–20% repeats (Epplen et al., 1978, Burt, 2002, Schmid et al., 2002).

Three Cot fractions i.e. HR (highly repetitive), MR (middle repetitive), and SL (single/low-copy), based on the re-association kinetics of chicken genomic DNA were identified. The Cot curve of the chicken genome is a two-component curve, with a highly repetitive component with a $Cot_{1/2}$ of roughly 1 and a low-copy component with a $Cot_{1/2}$ of ~1000 (Epplen et al. 1978). The MR fraction represents sequences reannealing between Cot 10 and Cot 100, thus spanning the gap in the chicken Cot curve between the least repetitive HR sequences and the most repetitive SL. Because the MR fraction is an ad hoc rather than a specific Cot component, it lacks a true $Cot_{1/2}$.

The repetitive DNA fraction, sometimes referred to as "junk DNA," includes short tandem repeats (e.g., telomeric and centromeric repeats) as well as numerous families of interspersed repeats that are often derived from transposable elements. Transposable elements are subdivided on the basis of whether their mobility involves an mRNA intermediate (Class 1) or the DNA itself (Class 2). Class 1 elements are further subdivided on the basis of the presence or absence of long terminal repeats (LTR). Class 1 non-LTR retrotransposons are also referred to as long and short interspersed nuclear elements (LINEs and SINEs), respectively. It has been speculated that the relatively small genome size of birds in general, and chickens in particular, may reflect selective pressure to optimize metabolism and to minimize the amount of repetitive DNA (Gregory 2002). The most abundant DNA elements known in the chicken genome to date are non-LTR retrotransposons of the *CR1* family, present in an estimated 100,000 copies and six distinct subfamilies of *CR1* (*CR1-A* through *CR1-F*) have been identified (Vandergon and Reitman 1994).

Another major repeat class populating the chicken genome is short tandem repeats. One example is the telomeric repeat, which consists of tandem arrays of many thousands of copies of the short sequence motif AATGGG. Compared with other vertebrates, chicken chromosomes contain large amounts of telomeric DNA and comprise 3%–4% of the genome (Delaney et al. 2003). Centromeres and subtelomeric regions also contain multiple classes of larger tandemly repeated units. The most abundant repeat type found in chicken is *CNM* (Matzke et al. 1990), a tandem repeat with a unit size of <40 bp. *CNM* repeats are members of a large superfamily that also includes other tandem repeats such as *PIR* (Wang et al. 2002) and *XhoI* (Klein and Ellendorf 2000). They show structural and sequence similarity with *CNM* repeats and are therefore believed to share a common ancestor.

Genome organization in guinea fowl: Very preliminary studies have been done regarding genome organization. Restriction enzyme profiles are useful in identifying species specific difference in DNA organization. The repetitive DNA sequence when cut with a restriction enzyme yield discrete bands because of their high copy number against a uniform smear of fluorescence. In guinea fowl, the extracted genomic DNA was digested with 15 restriction enzymes i.e. enzymes were tested, out of which 5 were tetra cutter (Table 7.2). The complete digestion of genomic DNA has resulted in a continuous smear from the 23 kb fragment to below 560 bp. No discrete bands

Table 7.2 : Restriction enzyme profile of guinea fowl with different restriction enzymes

Enzyme	Type of cutter	Restriction profile	Enzyme	Type of cutter	Restriction profile
Hae III	Tetra cutter	S	Hpa II	Tetra cutter	S
Mbo I	Tetra cutter	S	Msp I	Tetra cutter	S
Taq I	Tetra cutter	S	Apa I	Hexa cutter	S + FB
Dra I	Hexa cutter	S + FB	Ecor I	Hexa cutter	S + FB
Ecor V	Hexa cutter	S	Hinc II	Hexa cutter	S
Hind III	Hexa cutter	S + FB	Hinf I	Hexa cutter	S
Nde I	Hexa cutter	S + FB	Pst I	Hexa cutter	S + FB
Sac I	Hexa cutter	S + FB			

were observed with any of the enzymes (Fig 7.2). No genotype or sex difference could be observed in restriction digestion profile from these three poultry populations. The repetitive DNA sequence when cut with a restriction enzyme yield discrete bands because of their high copy number against a uniform smear of fluorescence. The absence of any discrete bands in present study on restriction digestion with all the restriction enzymes suggest that the satellite DNA appears to have a little proportion of the total genomic DNA in guinea fowl. In other domestic poultry species, similar pattern is reported. In general, it may be concluded that only a small fraction of the total genomic DNA is present as satellite DNA in all the

domesticated poultry species and the restriction enzyme analysis of repetitive satellite DNA sequence is not a potential method for finding the genetic markers in poultry species including guinea fowl (Sharma et al., 1999).

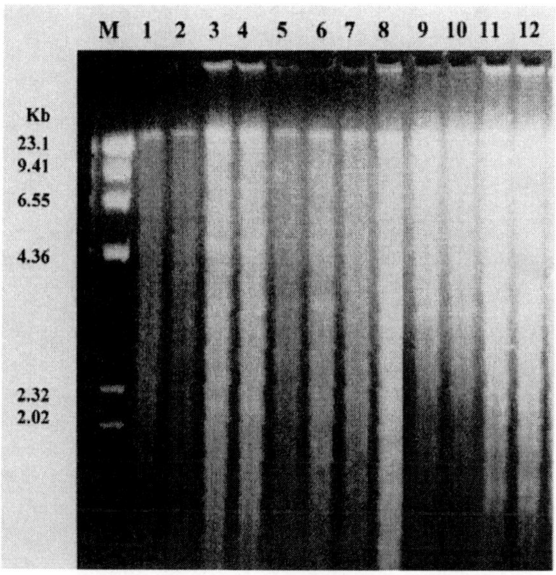

Fig. 7.2 : Restriction enzyme profile of guinea fowl with Hind *III*. Pearl: Lane 1-4, Lavender: Lane 5-8, White: Lane 9-12. M : Molecular size marker (l DNA digested with Hind *III*)

Sequence variability

It is quite evident that a huge amount of genetic variation exists in all eukaryotic genome. The assaying this genetic variation through some protocol has developed the concept of molecular marker. Hence, a genetic or molecular marker is a site of heterozygosity for some type of neutral DNA variation. Neutral variations are that which are not associated with any measurable phenotypic variation. Such DNA locus or fragments are called genetic/ DNA marker. There are several types of DNA markers and these markers can be classified into two types i.e. Type I and Type II. While Type I markers are associated with a gene of known function, Type II markers seems to have association with anonymous gene segments of one sort or another.

DNA-based markers could alternatively be grouped into clone/sequence based (CSB) markers and fingerprint (FP) markers (Dodgson *et al.*, 1997). The first category requires the isolation of a cloned DNA fragment and often determination of some, if not all of its DNA sequence. The CSB markers include microsatellites, RFLP, STS and EST among others. The FP markers require no prior knowledge of the sequence of the polymorphic region or isolation of a cloned DNA fragment and they include RAPD, VNTRs, AFLP, RLGS and many others. The FP markers are inherently Type II markers, whereas, CSB markers include both Type I and Type II markers. Of the CSB markers, microsatellite markers are predominant markers and are more commonly used for genome mapping, detection of polymorphism among individuals, estimation of genetic similarity/ relatedness among and within populations.

Further, markers may be random or specific. The markers which detect the sequence variability at one or more loci, but do not able to give the location of this variability are random markers. The VNTRs and RAPD are the good example of random markers. The specific markers, detects the sequence variability in a known region e.g. Microsatellite or Simple Sequence Repeat (SSR) markers.

Random Genetic polymorphism among guinea fowl varieties

Guinea fowl varieties, though different in plumage pattern, did not differ for their productive performance much. Hence the randomly amplified polymorphic DNA (RAPD) markers were used to detect polymorphism between as well as within the guinea fowl varieties and this polymorphism was further used to estimate genetic similarity within as well as between the varieties. A total of 32 decamer primers viz., OPA-1, 2, 3, 5, 6, 7, 9, 10 and 11; OPB-19; OPI-5; OPP-1 to 10 and OPM-1 to 11 (Operon Technologies, Inc., Almeda,

California) were used and only 12 of these yielded distinct amplification profile (Fig. 7.3). Number of amplification products varied from 14 to 24 with a size range of 250 to 4000 bp. However, varieties were not found to differ for average number of fragments resolved per primer. A total of 166 fragments were amplified and 27 (17%) of these showed polymorphism. The number of polymorphic loci detected by each primers ranged from 1 to 7, however, average number of the polymorphic loci per primer was more or less similar (2.1-2.7) in the three varieties of guinea fowl (Sharma et al., 1998).

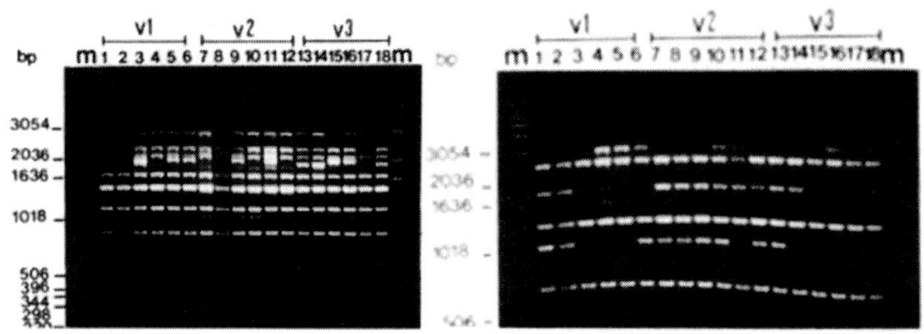

Fig. 7.3 : RAPD profiles in three varieties of guinea fowl generated by different random primers. V1: Pearl, V2: Lavender, V3: White

The RAPD polymorphism was used in estimating the infra and inter varietal genetic variation in three varieties of guinea fowl (Lavender, Pearl and White) The estimates, measured as band sharing were high for within population (0.946-0.971) and between population (0.990-0.999) genetic similarity. The respective estimates were 0.898-0.929 and 0.923-0.928 when estimated as frequency of occurrence of bands. The results indicated a very low level of intra and inter varietal genetic variation in these guinea fowl varieties, which in turn suggested the low level of genetic variation in these populations. The possible reasons for this high genetic similarity were evolution from small base and closed flock mating.

Sequence variability in genes influencing disease resistance

I. Major Histocompatability Complex genes

The Major Histocompatability Complex (MHC) is defined as the molecules displayed on cells surfaces and are involved in "Antigen presentation" and lymphocytes recognition. They control the immune response through recognition of "self" and "non-self" and consequently, serve as targets in transplantation rejection. The human MHC is a group of several genes which are present on chromosome 6. While BCA region codes for Class I molecules, class II molecules are encoded by D region. An intermediate region between the BCA and D encodes class III molecules as well as several complement components.

Avian Major Histocompatibility complex

Initially, the chicken MHC was described as a blood group locus (Briles *et al.* 1950). Schierman and Nordskog (1961) identified MHC *B* complex in chickens by the ability of leukocytes to give strong graft rejection and chicken was the second in whom MHC was identified. High polymorphism exhibited by some MHC loci is the most important feature of the chicken MHC and these loci are considered to be the most polymorphic among the MHCs in animals. In chicken, the MHC is located on 16th chromosome, which is medium sized micro-chromosome (Goto *et al.*, 1988).

Kauffman *et al.*, (1999) described the structure of chicken MHC and found it 20 fold smaller than human MHC as the core region i.e. the proper MHC (B) is only 92 kb long and contains 19 genes (Fig 7.4) making the chicken MHC remarkably compact, but to possess all essential MHC genes found in mammalian MHC. The chicken MHC has three regions i.e. Class I, II and III. The class III region is located outside the class II and class I regions. The region from the class II (B-L) b genes to the class I (B-F) a genes is especially compact and do not has repetitive elements or repeats. Total eleven genes present in this 44 kb region have average intron sizes of 200 nucleotides. It makes this region to be as little as one-third of the size of mammalian counterparts.

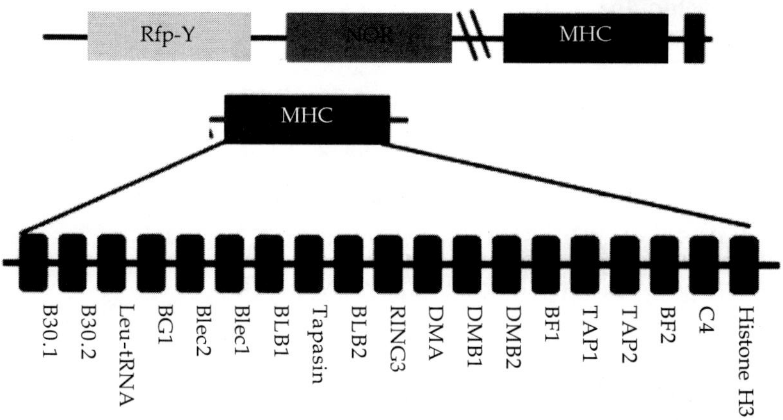

Fig. 7.4 : Diagrammatic presentation of MHC in chicken

Extensive cloning and sequencing of the different regions of the chicken MHC has confirmed that chicken MHC is comprised of three chromosomal regions or loci namely BF, BL and BG (Bourlet et al., 1988; Goto et al., 1988; Guillemot et al., 1988). While BF and BL produces class I and class II antigens respectively, the BG region produces class IV antigen. These three loci possess strong linkage as no recombination between the B-F and B-L loci have been reported (Guillemot et al., 1988), however, several recombinations between the B-G and B-F as well as BG and BL have been observed (Hala et al., 1981).

A nomenclature for B and Y (*Rfp-Y*) loci and alleles has been developed (Miller *et al.*, 2004). Guillemot *et al.* (1988) produced the first molecular map of the chicken MHC, locating class I, class II, and additional linked loci in four cosmid contigs (CC1, CC2, CC3, and CC4). Subsequently, contigs CC2, CC3, and CC4, were mapped to a separate gene region called *Y (Rfp-Y)*. Sequencing of CC1 locates two class I (BF1 and BF2) and two class II (BLBI and BLB2) loci amid 15 other genes and resulted in recognition that B is small, comparatively simple and densely packed with genes (Kaufman *et al.*, 1999).

MHC Class I genes

The Classical structure of Class I molecules has two polypeptide chains i.e. an α chain or heavy chain, which id coded by MHC and a β chain, known as beta-2 microglobulin i.e. β2m, encloded by non-MHC gene (Fig 7.5). The α chain or heavy chain is comprised of five domains, among which N or α1, C1 or α2 and C2 or α3 are extracellular domains.

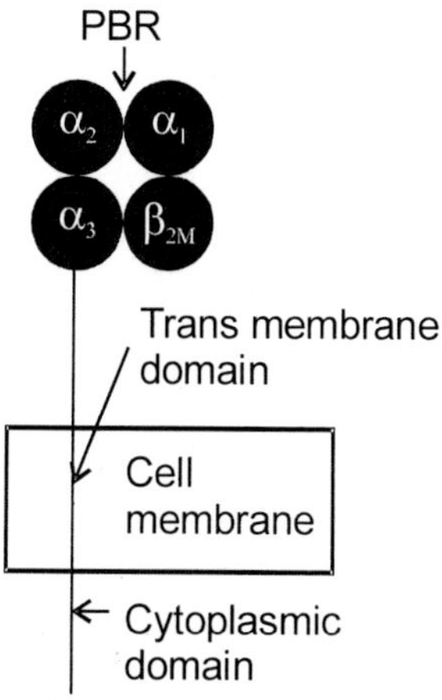

Fig. 7.5 : The MHC class 1 molecule has three globular domains α1, α2 and α3. The α3 domain is closely associated with the non-MHC-encoded β2M. There is transmembrane and a cytoplasmic domain

Other two domains are one trans-membrance domain, where the polypeptode chain passes through the plasma membrane and other cytoplasmic domain present in cell cytoplasm. A groove, known as peptide-binding region (PBR) is formed by α1 and α2 domains. The PBR has a floor of 8 stranded β pleated sheet with two opposite walls consisting of parallel strands of an α helix. While α1 domain contributes 4 strands of β pleated sheet and one α helix, remaining 4 strands of β pleated sheet and one α helix was contributed by α2 domain. The PBR region exhibit high variability in amino acids sequence as this region interacts with amino acids in the peptide fragments. This genetic variability among the class I MHC products results in variation in the chemical surface of the peptide binding groove. For binding of a peptide, one or more specific amino acids at a fixed position, frequently either terminal or penultimate position is required. Other polymorphic residues of the MHC molecule are those in contact with the T cell receptor (TCR), which interacts with both peptide and the MHC molecules itself. The $\alpha3$ domain is highly conserved and is homologus to Ig constant domains and non-covalently bound to $\beta2m$, an invariant molecule, also homologous to Ig constant domains. The $\alpha3$ domain and $\beta2m$ interacts with $\alpha1$ and $\alpha2$ domains to maintain their proper confirmation. The $\alpha3$ domain has a binding site for CD8, which is expressed on cytolytic T cells that recognizes class I MHC molecules.

The two class I loci described variously in the literature and in GenBank. The BFI locus has been called B-FI, B-F minor, and BFa2. The BF2 locus has been called B-FIV, B-F major, and B-FI (complex hybridization data resulted in the earlier mistaken inclusion of two additional loci, B-FII and BFIII, on the original map) (Guillemot *et al.* 1988; Kaufman *et al.* 1999). The BF2 locus is predominantly expressed; hence, this locus has been referred to as *B-F major,* with the less well-expressed *BF1* locus described as *B-F minor. BFI* and *BF2* are similar to classical

MHC class I genes in other species bearing identifiers derived from species-specific nomenclatures, such as *HLA-A, HLA-B* and *HLA-C* in man, and *H2-K, H2-D,* and *H2-L* in mouse, and the *RTI Al, A2,* and *A3* genes in rat, as well as numerous classical class I genes identified in other species that bear identifiers suggested in the unifying nomenclature proposed in 1990 (Klein *et al.* 1990). The two class IIâ loci within CCI (Guillemot *et al.*, 1988) now termed BLB1 and BLB2 contain genes that are related to the class II (3-chain genes identified within the D region in the human and many other mammalian MHC, mouse H2AN and H2-Ebl loci and the DB loci in other bird species, including, quail (Kulski *et al.*, 2002), pheasant (Wittzell *et al.*, 1999), etc.

NumeMHC I gene

The NumeMHC I amino acid sequence was 189 amino acids in size, comprising of 10 amino acid of signal peptide (partial), 90 amino acids in a_1 domain (complete exon 2) and 89 amino acids in a_2 domain (partial exon 3). In guinea fowl, the a_1 domain had 90 aa in size against the 88 aa in chicken, duck and goose, however, in quail, it had 90 aa. Similarly, in guinea fowl, the a_2 domain was partial and 89 amino acids. While in chicken and quail it is 91 amino acids in size, duck and goose had 92 aa in a_2 domain (Singh et al., 2010a).

Structural homology of NumeMHC I: Sequence alignment with mammalian MHC showed that many of the conserved features of mammalian MHC class I glycoprotein was conserved in guinea fowl (Fig 7.6). Two disulphide binding cysteines at 101 and 164 positions in a_2 domain and a potential N-glycosylation site at 87 position in a_1 domain were conserved. All the conserved residues interacting with the amino terminus of the bonds peptide in the HLA/H2 PBS i.e. Y^7, Y^{59}, Y^{159} and Y^{171} were also conserved in guinea fowl also i.e. Y^7, Y^{60}, Y^{159} and Y^{171}. Three of the four conserved residues, which interact with the carboxyl terminus of the peptides in HLA/H2 i.e. T^{143}, K^{146} and W^{146} were also conserved in guinea fowl i.e. T^{142}, K^{145} and W^{146}. However, the residue Y^{84} was not conserved and replaced by R^{85} in guinea fowl. This overall conservation was also reported in MHC I sequences from other poultry species such as duck, goose and in other birds also (Singh, 2009).

In chicken, a total of 20 presumed sites in a_1 domain and 16 presumed sites in a_2 domain were identified, which interacts with peptide

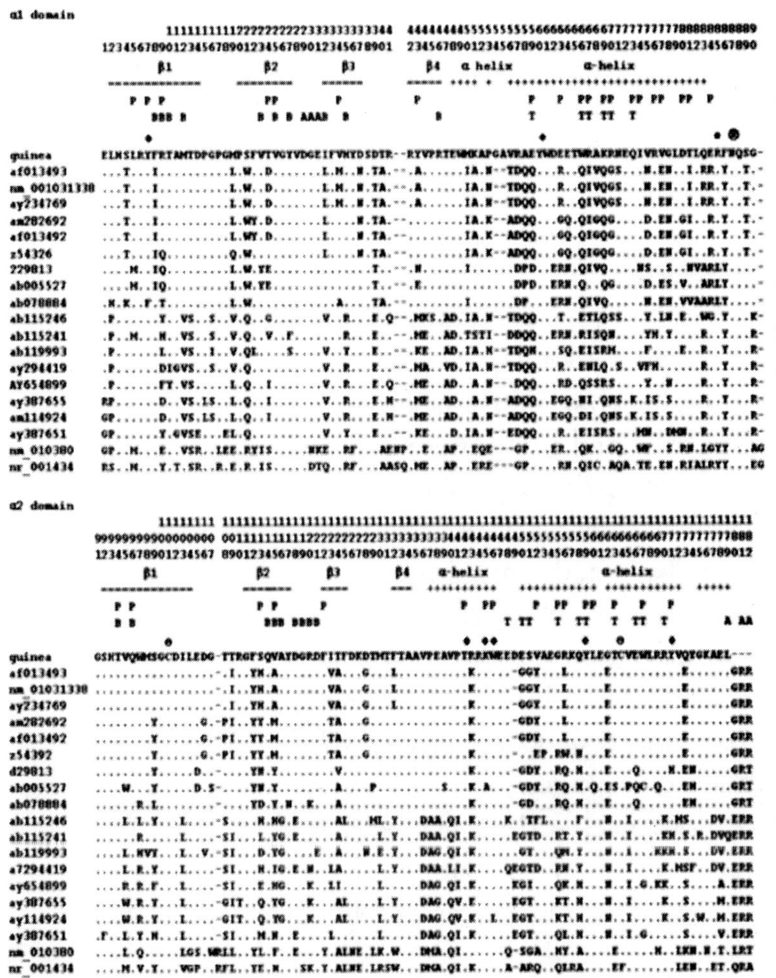

Fig. 7.6 : Alignment of the translated amino acid sequences of the a1 domains of MHC class I molecules from guinea fowl, other poultry species, mouse and human. "-" : gaps in the sequences; "." same amino acid as in guinea fowl, = : beta strand; + : alpha helix; P : presumed contacts with peptides; A : presumed contacts with alpha3 domain; B : contacts with beta microglobulin, T : presumed contacts with T cell receptor; ¨ and • : conserved and not conserved key amino acids which interacts with antigenic peptide terminal in HLA-A2, respectively; ? : conserved cysteins for disulphide bonds, ® : conserved N-glycosylation site.

(Kaufman *et al.*, 1992). In guinea fowl, 13 sites (65 %) in a_1 domain and 4 sites (25 %) in a_2 domain showed amino acid substitutions. In a_1 domain, 32 amino acids are involved in b strands, while 33 amino acids form the a-helix. The a-helix showed much higher amino acid variability (31.25 – 50.00 %) in comparison to b strands (60.61 – 69.70 %) between guinea fowl and other poultry species. Lima-Rosa *et al.* (2004) also observed the higher amino acid variability in and around the a-helix region in chicken. In a_2 domain, 27 amino acids are involved in b strand, while 37 amino acids forms the a-helix. In a_2 domain, though more or less similar trend was observed, but the amount of amino acid variability (25 – 44 % in a-helix and 22 – 54 % in b strands) was much lower as compared to a_1 domain. In guinea fowl, the addition of two amino acids in a_1 domain and one amino acid in a_2 domain was in highly variable -helix region, hence do not seem to influence the function of the peptide binding region.

Phylogenetic analysis: Phylogenetic tree, based on pair wise genetic distances estimated on the amino acid variability in a_1 and a_2 domains revealed two major clusters, comprising of guinea fowl, quail and chicken in one, while duck and goose in other. In first cluster, guinea fowl make separate branch, while chicken and quails are clustered together. In other clusters, goose and duck cluster together, except one goose sequence, which make a separate branch. In the lineage of MHC class I molecules, guinea fowl showed more closeness to the chicken and quail, while the duck and goose seemed to have a distant lineage.

MHC Class II gene

The MHC class II molecule contains two non-covalently associated polypeptide chains i.e. a chain and b chain and both are MHC encoded and polymorphic. Each chain has two domains i.e. a_1 and a_2 for á chain; and b_1 and $_2$ for b chain (Fig 7.7). The peptide-binding region is formed by the interaction of the a_1 and b_1 domains. There is a groove having a floor of 8 b pleated sheets and two "walls" with a helices. The a_1 and b_1 domains make equal contribution of 4 b pleated sheets and one a helix to this structure. The amino acids facing the groove showed maximum variability. The genetic polymorphism determines the chemical structure of the groove and influences the specificity and affinity of peptide binding and T cell recognition. Peptides associated with class II MHC are 13-15 amino acids long, the longer peptides projects from the ends of the groove. Anchor sites for one or more amino acids exist in the groove, but these occur at more variable locations. The immunoglobulin like region formed by a_2 and b_2 domains is folded into Ig like domains. These are largely non-polymorphic. The correlation of CD4 expression on helper T cells with a specific TCR for class II MHC molecules is due to binding of the CD4 molecules to the Ig like non-polymorphic b_2 domain of class II molecules.

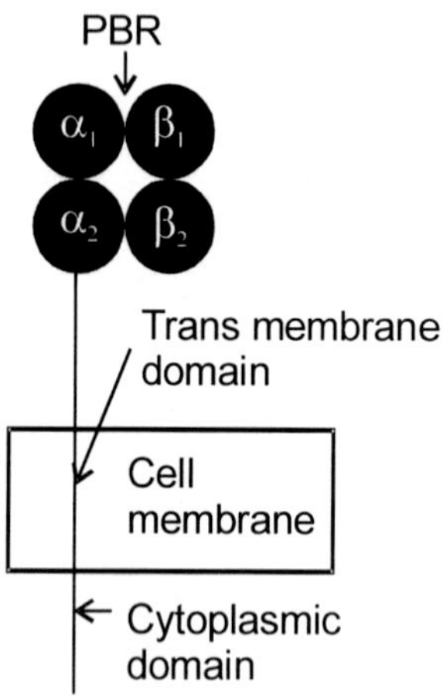

Fig. 7.7 : MHC class II molecules comprise two non-identical peptides (α and β) which are non-covalently associated alongwith trans-memberane and one cytoplasmic domains. Peptide binding region is formed by interaction α_1 and β_1).

The B-L region codes for genes, which produce class II antigens. Five class II (B-L) B genes were reported to be encoded in the major histocompatibility complex (MHC) of chickens of the B^{12} haplotype (Zoorob *et al.*, 1990). On the basis of sequence similarities B-L BI and B-L BII genes belongs to one isotype family (B–L BII family) characterized by 97% sequence identity in the protein coding region in the standard B12 haplotypes. The B–L BIII , B-L BIV and B-L BV genes belongs to the B-L B III family and share 99% protein coding sequence identity with each other. The B–L b III family genes are 82% similar to genes in the B –L b family (Zoorab *et. al.*, 1993). The B-L BI and B-L BII are the predominantly expressed B-L B genes among the five such genes described in chickens of the B^{12} haplotyps (Phar et al, 1993). Subsequent studies showed that BLBII is highly polymorphic and has been widely studied in different avian species (Wittzell *et al.* 1999, Hosomichi *et al.* 2006, Ahmed et al. 2007).

NumeMHC Class II gene in guinea fowl

In guinea fowl, the size of b_1 and b_2 domains was 89 and 93 amino acids. The b_1 domain was found to be highly variable in guinea fowl. Highly polymorphic nature of b_1 domain was also reported in other poultry species like chicken, quail and duck (Singh et al., 2010b).

Structural homology: Sequence homology comparison of the b_1 and b_2 domains in guinea fowl with the respective domains from other poultry species as well with human MHC (Fig 7.8 and 7.9) showed conservation at various important sites in guinea fowl

```
β1 Domain
                                  ↓________________________________________________________↓
                                   1111111111222222222233333333334444444444555555555566666666667777777777888888888
                          12345678901234567890123456789012345678901234567890123456789012345678901234567890123456789
                            = = = =   ===   =  = =     =  ======     =   =       ==   =======  = ===  =         =
Numida-meleagris-1        FFQYSFIGECHFLNGTERVRFMHRYIYNRQEYTHYDSDVGKFVADTALGERQAEHYNSNTEYMEYLQGEPDRFCRHNYGVGESFTVQRR
Numida-meleagris-2        ....GVRF............LVD.Q......FM.F......Y....P...P...Y....P.IL.D.MNAV.T..Y....L.........
Numida-meleagris-3        ....GVRF.........Q..LVA.Q.....QFM.F......Y....P...P...Y......LL.D.MNRV.AA..YT...L.........
Numida-meleagris-4        ...W.LRA...Y......M.LVA.Q......F..F......Y...AP...P........P.IL.NQMNQV.T........L.......S
Numida-meleagris-5        ...W.LRA...Y......M.LVA.Q......F..F......Y...AP...P........P.IL.NQMNQV.T........L.......-
Gallus-gallus-1           ..FCGA.F...Y........YLQ.......QLV.F..........P...P...YW...A.LL.NIMNIA.GS......IL.......S
Gallus-gallus-2           ...WT.KA...Y......A..LE.H.....QFM.F......Y....P.......IW...A.IL.DEMNAV.T...............S
Gallus-gallus-3           ..FRGM.Y...Y........LLD.Q.....QTS.F......Y....P...P...YW...A.F..IKRN.V..V.......V.......S
Gallus-gallus-4           ..F.GA.....Y........YLD.E.....Q.A.F..........P...P...YW...G.LL.N.MNIA.GP......IL.......S
Coturnix-coturnix-1       Y..H...S.........Q...LVD.......Q...F......Y....P.......YW..Q..IL.DARDAV.TY..Y....D.P.....S
Coturnix-coturnix-2       Y..H...S.........Q...LVD.......Q...F......Y....P.......YW..Q..IL.DARDAV.TY..Y....D.P.....S
Coturnix-coturnix-3       Y..FYARS..Q...D......VVG......Q...F..........P...L.......Q...L..TR.AV.TY.......F..I....S
Coturnix-coturnix-4       ...HT................VV.......Q...F...L.......P....P..YW..D..E...RRN.V.T.........F.......S
Phasianus-colchicus-1     ..LHGV.F....V...QQ..HVE.D.H...Q.A.F......Y....P...L...YW.N........RR..V..Y.....EGV........
Phasianus-colchicus-2     ..LHGV.F....V...QQ..HVE.D.H...Q.A.F......Y....P...L...YW.N........RR..V..Y.....EGV........
Phasianus-colchicus-3     ..LDGV.F....V...QQ..HVE.D.....QLL.F......Y....P...L...YW.N........RR..V..Y......F........
Phasianus-colchicus-4     ..Y..TTS....Q....QI..LD..F....QF..F..........P...PV..QW....QTL..AR.AV.WY.....EGV........
Anas-platyrhynchos-1      ..HEMLAF...Y.....Q..YLE.H.....QFMQF.....H.....E..KPL.DNW..RP.IL.DRR.SV.TY..R..NLVTP...D..
Anas-platyrhynchos-2      ...LMLVF..QY........LLE.D.....QFM.......RY.V..E..KPI.DYL..QP.IL.QRRAAV.-T.....E.SD.YILR.K
Anas-platyrhynchos-3      ...FLGTC...Y........YLDT......Q.A.F.....HY....E..KPD.DYW..QP.IL..QR.SV........E.SDTYILH..
Homo-sapiens              R.LWQPKR....F.........LD..F..QE.SVRF.....E.R.V.E..RPD..YW..QKDIL.QARAAV.TY.......V........
```

Fig. 7.8 : Alignment of the translated amino acid sequences of the a1 domains of MHC class I molecules from guinea fowl, other poultry species, mouse and human. "-" : gaps in the sequences; "." same amino acid as in guinea fowl, = : beta strand; + : alpha helix; P : presumed contacts with peptides; A : presumed contacts with alpha3 domain; B : contacts with beta microglobulin, T : presumed contacts with T cell receptor; ¨ and • : conserved and not conserved key amino acids which interacts with antigenic peptide terminal in HLA-A2, respectively; ? : conserved cysteins for disulphide bonds, Ò : conserved N-glycosylation site.

β_2 Domain

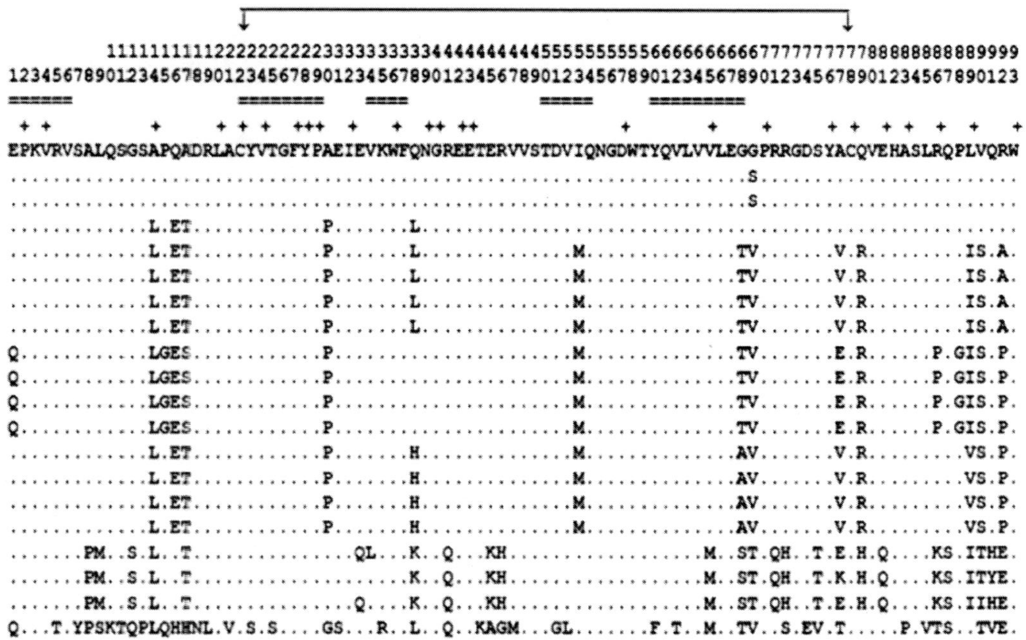

Fig. 7.9 : Alignment of the translated amino acid sequences of the b_2 domains of MHC molecules class II from guinea fowl, other poultry species, mouse and human. "-" : gaps in the sequences; "." same amino acid as in guinea fowl, = : residues involved in formation of b strand; + : residues commonly found in immunoglobulin like regions

(Singh et al., 2010c). Among different residues, the most important were cysteins at 10th (C^{10}) and 74th (C^{74}) positions in b_1 domain and at 22nd and 78th positions in b2 domain involved in formation of disulphide bonds and N-glycosylation (NGT at positions 14-16) sites in b_1 domain and these sites were perfectly conserved in guinea fowl. These Csyteins were also reported to be conserved in different poultry species including chicken. Residues FDSDVG (at 35-40) and charged pair (R^{20+} D^{38-}) conserved in most of avian species were also conserved in guinea fowl. In b_1 domain, 34 residues are thought to be involved in the tertiary conformation of the antigen binding domain in HLA-A2 and 58.33 % of these were conserved in guinea fowl. In other poultry species, similar proportion of conserved residues at this region sites were observed. Similarly in b_2 domain, 32 residues were assumed to be involved in the formation of b strand of the immunoglobulin like region in HLA-A2 and 65.63 % of these were conserved in guinea fowl. In other poultry species, similar proportions of conserved residues were observed.

The between species genetic distances, estimated as Poisson correction using the cumulative amino acid variability in b_1 domain and b_2 domain revealed lower but similar genetic distances between guinea fowl with chicken, quail and pheasant, whereas with duck, it was high. Singh *et al.* (2005) also observed that the duck showed much lower genetic similarity with other avian species (55.5-61.1 %), while these poultry species showed high and similar magnitude of genetic similarity (67.00-78.7 %) among themselves in b_1 domain.

The phylogenetic tree clearly revealed that the avian MHC sequences clustered together and among avian sequences, clustering is largely by species wise. The species wise clustering might be due to species specific residues (Takahashi & Nei, 2000) and such patterns of the sequences may be explained by gene conversion and balancing selection (Edwards *et al.*, 1999; Miller and Lambert, 2004). Among avian species, the duck MHC are clustered separately suggesting its separate evolution. Xia *et al.* (2004) found that duck MHC class I clusters quite distantly from chicken MHC. The guinea fowl made a separate branch, though within the first major cluster not showing more closeness with any one of the other poultry species i.e. chicken, quail and pheasant. Ahmed *et al.* (2007) studied the phylogenetic relationship between turkey MHC with other avian as well as mammalian MHC and found that avian MHC sequences clustered together, separated from the mammalian sequences by a long branch. Avian sequences clustered largely by species, although there were some patterns consistent with orthologous loci.

II. Cytokines

Cytokines are proteins or peptides secreted by the cells that play a key role in immune and inflammatory responses through activation and regulation of other cells and tissues.

Until recently, only a limited number of immune regulator and effector genes and their encoded polypeptides were identified in avian species due to the low level of sequence homologies with their mammalian counterparts. Among these, the cytokines are essential effector molecules of innate and adaptive immunity against pathogenic microorganisms. Current dogma holds that cytokines are classified by the Thl-Th2 paradigm according to their role in the immune response (Mosmann *et al.*, 1986; Mosmann & Coffman, 1989 & Degen *et al.*, 2005).

As in mammals, host inflammation and innate immunity in chickens are mediated by Th1 or Th1-related cytokines, including interferon (IFN)-á, -â and –g, IL-1â, IL-2, IL-6, IL-10, IL-12, IL-15, IL-16, IL-17 and IL-18. In addition, other molecules such as myeloid differentiation factor 88 (MyD88), TNF receptor associated factor-5 (TRAF-5), and inducible nitric oxide synthase (iNOS) are involved in the Th1 inflammatory response to avian pathogens (Lin *et al.*, 1996 & Caldwell *et a1.*, 2005). The Th2 or Th2-related molecules, classically defined as driving humoral immunity, produce a distinct panel of cytokines, in particular IL-3, IL-4, IL-5, IL-13, granulocyte macrophage-colony stimulating factor (GM-CSF), and transforming growth factor (TGF)-â4 (Jakowlew *et al.*, 1988 & Avery *et al.*, 2004).

Interferon-g (IFN-g) gene analysis

Total size of gf-IFN-g was 498 bp against the 495 bp in all other poultry species and this increase in size was due to insertion of three nucleotides at 191, 192 and 193 nucleotide positions in guinea fowl. The gf-IFN-g amino acid sequence comprised of 165 aa, while in other poultry species, it was 164 aa. An additional amino acid 'Serine' was found at 66th amino acid position. The change in amino acid profile at this position is an important change and needs to be studied for its influence on protein structure and function of IFN-g in guinea fowl (Goyal et al., 2008a).

The exon-intron structure of IFN-g showed considerable similarity in organization with mammals and aves (Kaiser et al., 1998b). The gene comprises four exons. The first exon contains 5′ UTR and 123 nucleotides which codes for the signal sequence of 19 amino acid and the first 22 amino acid of the mature protein. Exons 2 and 3 comprised of 69 and 180 nucleotides, coding for 23 and 60 aa, respectively. Exon 4 comprised of 120 nucleotides coding for 40 aa, 3 nucleotides of stop codon and the 3′ UTR (>1278 bp). Within chicken, the nucleotide sequences as well as amino acid sequences were highly conserved. The highly conserved structure of the gene and high degree of overall identity at the predicted primary amino acid sequence level of protein was reported among these species (Kaiser *et al.*, 1998).

Though guinea fowl showed the polymorphism of more or less similar magnitude with all other galliformes in term of absolute polymorphism, but the proportion of the non-synonymous nucleotide substitutions was much low between guinea fowl and chicken as evident from the ratio between non- synonymous to synonymous nucleotide substitutions, which, was lowest (1.5:1) between guinea fowl and chicken. Between guinea fowl and pheasant, quail as well as turkey, it was 3.1:1 to 3.2:1, while between guinea fowl and duck as well as goose, it was 3.8:1 to 4.1:1. These comparisons suggest that most of the changes in the IFN-g sequences did not cause the change in amino acids, hence were synonymous (Fig 7.10).

Phylogenetic analysis: Preliminary phylogenetic analysis showed that all the IFN-g sequences from galliformes species have been clustered together and separated from the anseriformes sequences, which formed another cluster. Within galliformes cluster, guinea fowl sequence has been placed separately. While all chicken sequences were in one group, turkey and pheasant sequences in another group and quail in separate group.

Inducible Nitric Oxide synthase (iNOS) gene analysis

A ~792 bp fragment of iNOS was amplified in guinea fowl (Goyal et al., 2008b). The iNOS amino acid sequence comprised of 263 amino acids in guinea fowl. The comparable sequence from chicken also produced 263 aa, where as in quail, the

```
                     1 1111111112 2222222223 3333333334 4444444445 5555555556 6666666667 7777777778 888
              1234567890 1234567890 1234567890 1234567890 1234567890 1234567890 1234567890 1234567890 123
GF1           MTCQTYNLFV LSVIMIYFGR TANSLNLAQL EDDIDKLKAD FNSSHSDVAD GGPIFIEKLK NWTGQSNEKK IILSQIVSMY LEM
GF2           .......... .......... .......... .......... .......... .......... .......... .......... ...
GF3           .......... .......... .......... .......... .......... .......... .......... .......... ...
DQ470471-ch   .......... .......Y.H ..S....V.. Q......... .......... ....IV.... ...ER-...R .......... ...
AY705909-ch   .......... .......Y.H ..S....V.. Q......... .......... ....IV.... ...ER-...R .......... ...
AY501004-ch   .......... .......Y.H ..S....V.. Q......... .......... ....IV.... ...ER-...R .......... ...
AY163160      .......... .......Y.H ..S..I.V.. Q...A..... .......... ....IA.... ...ER-.Q.R .......... ...
AJ000725-tr   .......... .......Y.H ..S....V.. Q......... .......... ....IV.... ...ER-...R .......... ...
AF087134-dk   ......C... .........C SGSA.F.G.. QN........ ..A.N..... .N.V....V. ...ER-...R .......TL. ...
AF100929-dk   ......C... .........C SGSA.F.G.. QN........ ..A.N..... .N.V....V. ...ER-...R .......TL. ...
AJ001678-ql   .......... .......Y.H ..S....V.. Q......... .......... ....IV.... ...ER-...R .......... ...
AJ001289-ph   .......... .......Y.H ..S....V.. Q......... .......... ....IV.... ...ER-...R .......... ...

                    1111 1111111111 1111111111 1111111111 1111111111 1111111111 1111111111 111
              8888889999 9999990000 0000001111 1111112222 2222223333 3333334444 4444445555 5555556666 666
              4567890123 4567890123 4567890123 4567890123 4567890123 4567890123 4567890123 4567890123 456
GF1           FENTDQSKPH IKHISEELCT LRDSLSDGVK KVKDIMDLAK LQMTDLRIQR KAANELFIVL QKLVDPPSLK RKRNQPQRRC NC*
GF2           .......... .......... .......... .......... .......... .......... .....L.... .......... ...
GF3           .......... .......... .......... .......... .......... .......... .....L.... .......... ...
DQ470471-ch   L....K.... ........Y. .KNN.P.... .......... .P.N...... .......SI. ........F. ...S.S.... ...
AY705909-ch   L....K.... ........Y. .KNN.P.... .......... PP.N...... .......SI. ........F. ...S.S.... ...
AY501004-ch   L....K.... ........Y. .KNN.P.... .......... .P.N...... .......SI. ........F. ...S.S.... ...
AY163160      LA...KT... T.......Y. .KNN.P.... .......... .P.N...V.L .......SI. ....N...F. .NMS.S.... ...
AJ000725-tr   L....K.... ........Y. .KNN.P.... .......... ...N...... .......SI. ........S. ...SH..... ...
AF087134-dk   LKK..M.... ..NL..Q.N. ..NT..NDY. .FR.LVE.SN ..L.G.K... ..VS...S.. ....ETSTS. ...S.SPK.. R..
AF100929-dk   LKK..M.... ..NL..Q.N. ..NT..NDY. .FR.LVE.SN ..L.G.K... ..VS...S.. ....ETSTS. ...S.SPK.. R..
AJ001678-ql   L....K.... ........Y. .KNN.N..T. .......... ...N....H. ....D..S.. ........S. ...S.CL... S..
AJ001289-ph   L....K.... ........Y. .KNN.P.... .......... .R.N...... .......S.. ........S. ...S.S..K. ...
```

Fig. 7.10 : Amino acid sequence homology comparison between guinea fowl IFN-g and other poultry species available nucleotide sequence was partial and much smaller, hence produced only 123 amino acids. Out of 263 amino acids between guinea fowl and chicken, 7 (2.66 %) were polymorphic, while out of 123 amino acids between guinea fowl and quail, 4 (3.25 %) were polymorphic (Fig 7.11).

Phylogenetic analysis

Based on nucleotide sequence comparisons for iNOS gene, guinea fowl showed low and almost equal per cent divergence (3.9 – 4.6 %) with chicken and quail. Chicken and quail also showed very low per cent divergence (3.0 – 3.1 %) between them. The phylogenetic tree placed all the chicken sequences in one cluster and quail and guinea fowl as separate branches.

Interleukin 8 (IL-8)

A 578 bp fragment was amplified using the specific primers. No deletion or additions were observed in all the sequences, suggesting no size variation for IL8 CDS sequence among them. Sequence homology comparisons of GF with other poultry species revealed comparatively higher variations between GF & Goose and GF & Pigeon in comparison to that between GF & Chicken and GF & Turkey.

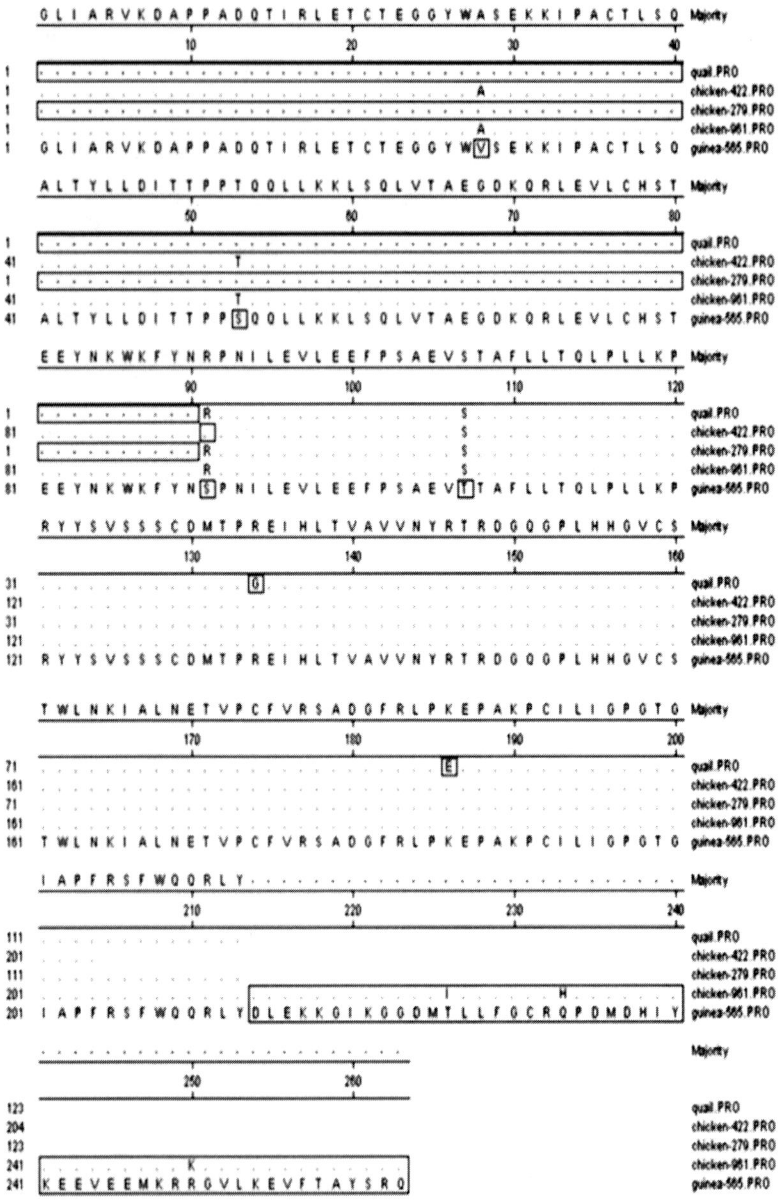

Fig. 7.11 : Amino acid sequence homology comparison between guinea fowl iNOS and other poultry species

Numbers of polymorphic sites were 17, 42, 18 and 48 between GF & Chicken, GF & Goose, GF & turkey and GF & Pigeon, yielding the percent polymorphism of 5.4, 13.5, 5.8 and 15.4 %, respectively.

The amino acid sequences of IL8 CDS from GF and other poultry species were aligned and studied for sequence homology (Fig 7.12). The aa sequence was 104 aa in size in GF as well as in all other poultry species. Number of polymorphic sites showing amino acid substitutions were 3,7, 4 and 11 between GF & Chicken, GF & Goose, GF & turkey and GF & Pigeon, yielding the percent polymorphism of 2.88, 6.73, 13.84 and 10.57 %, respectively. Among various amino acid substitutions between GF and different poultry species, G by S at 3 aa and V by I at 8 aa positions were important at these were specific to GF.

PCR-RFLP of BLB2 region in guinea fowl population diversified for immuno-competence and growth traits

Two resource populations i.e. one for high (HBW), medium (MBW) and low (LBW) body weight groups and other for high HA titre to SRBC (HA) and low HA titre to SRBC (LA) groups were used in PCR-RFLP analysis of b_1 domain of

```
                       1 1111111112 2222222223 3333333334
              1234567890 1234567890 1234567890 1234567890
GF            MNSKLGAILA LLLVSAALSQ GRTLVKMGNE LRCQCISTHS
CH-AJ009800   ..G....V.. .......... .......... ..........
CH-DQ393272   ..G....V.. .......... .......... ..........
GS-DQ3932774  ..G....V.. ...I.V.... ..S..R.... ..........
TR-DQ393276   ..G....V.. .......... .......... ..........
PG-DQ393275   ..G....V.. .F.I.V.V.. ....PR.AT. ......A...

              4444444445 5555555556 6666666667 7777777778
              1234567890 1234567890 1234567890 1234567890
GF            KFIHPKSIQD VKLTPSGPHC KNVEIIATLK DGREVCLDPT
CH-AJ009800   .......... .......... .......... ..........
CH-DQ393272   .......... .......... .......... ..........
GS-DQ3932774  .......... ....Q..... .......... .N........
TR-DQ393276   .......... .......... .......... .S........
PG-DQ393275   ...P..A... ....Q..... ....V..... ..........

                                  1 1111
              8888888889 9999999990 0000
              1234567890 1234567890 1234
GF            APWVQLIVKA LMAKAQLNSD APL*
CH-AJ009800   .......... .......... ....
CH-DQ393272   .......... .......... ....
GS-DQ3932774  .......... IL........ ....
TR-DQ393276   .......... .......... ....
PG-DQ393275   .....R..N. I......... ....
```

Fig. 7.12 : Amino acid sequence homology comparison between guinea fowl IL-8 CDS and other poultry species

BLB2 gene in guinea fowl. The restriction enzyme mapping of the 277 bp fragment of BLB2 gene revealed several restriction enzyme sites and among these, *Hae III* and *Taq I* were used for genotyping the resource populations in guinea fowl. In resource population, the mean body weight in high, medium and low body weight groups were 994.28±09.76, 914.00 ± 05.32 and 826.47±10.67, respectively and these body weight groups were significantly different with each other for 12 week of body weight. The *Hae* III as well as *Taq*I detected the polymorphism (Fig 7.13), but this PCR-RFLP was did not show any association with early body weight (Kumar et al., 2008).

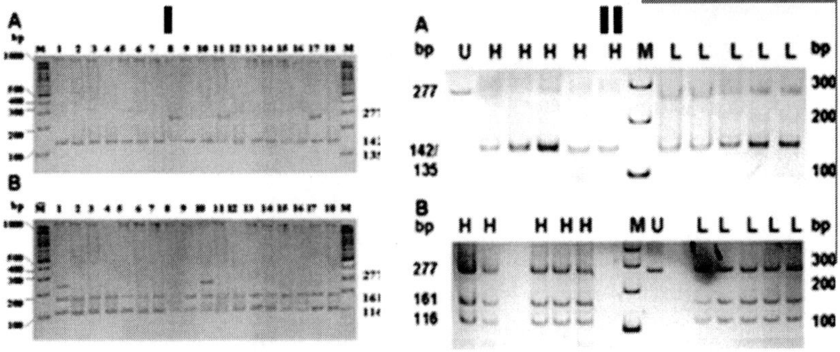

Fig. 7.13 : PCR-RFLP pattern with Hae III (A) and Taq I (B) restriction enzymes in I. body weight groups. High BW: 1-6; Medium BW: 7-12; Low BW: 13-18. M: 100 bp ladder; II. In HA titre groups, H: high HA titre; L: Low HA titre

Similarly, another resource population developed on the basis of antibody response to SRBC showed significant difference for HA titre in HA and LA groups. Only *Hae* III could detect polymorphism (Fig 7.14), but this PCR-RFLP pattern between HA and LA groups could not present any association with the antibody titre, suggesting that the nucleotide substitutions at 116 and 142 nt positions are not associated either with early body weight or antibody response to SRBC in guinea fowl (Kumar et al., 2008).

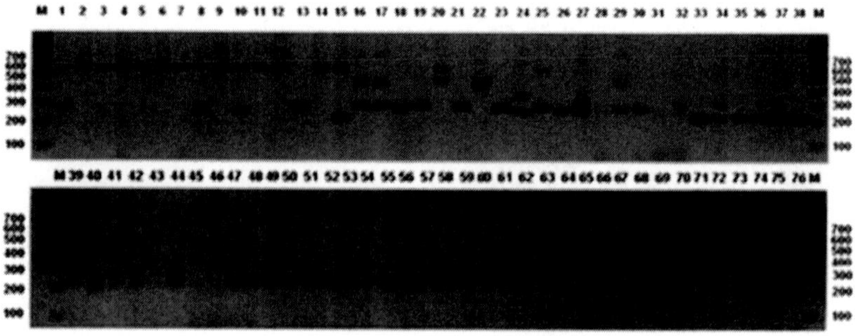

Fig. 7.14 : Allelic profile at LEI0258 loci in White Leghorn (1-15), Aseel (16-30), Kadaknath (31-45) and guinea fowl (46-76). M : 100 bp ladder

MHC Haplotyping in Guinea Fowl

For B haplotyping based on ADL0258 genotyping, a total of 76 guinea fowl birds of Lavender variety (GF) and 15 birds from each of the three chicken breeds i.e. White Leghorn (WL), Aseel (AS) and Red Cornish (RC) were genotyped. In microsatellite marker study in GF monomorphic pattern was observed and only 247 bp allele was found for LEI 258 locus suggesting presence of only one haplotype (Fig 7.14). However in chicken breeds, sizable polymorphism revealed presence of number of haplotype as already known (Gupta et al., 2008a).

In view of monomorphic pattern at LEI0258 locus, SSCP pattern for 277 bp fragment representing b1 domain of BLB 2 gene was studied. Presence of 6 SSCP patterns suggested the possibilities of more than one B haplotype in guinea fowl (Fig 7.15). The pattern

V was predominantly present in LHA and MHA groups, while completely absent in HHA group. Similarly, pattern IV showed maximum frequency in HHA (0.357), followed by MHA (0.200) and very low in LHA (0.053). The pattern III showed good frequency in all the groups (0.263 to 0.343). These preliminary trends are encouraging, but demands further investigation (Gupta et al., 2008b).

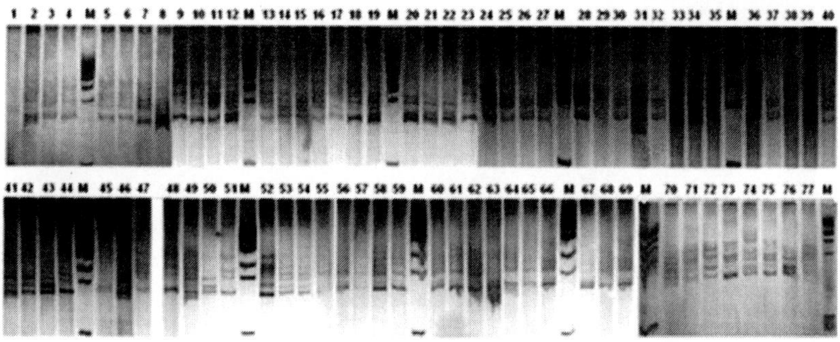

Fig. 7.15 : SSCP pattern in high HA titre (HHA), Medium HA titre (MHA) and Low HA titre (LHA) groups.

References

Ahmed, K.A., Saxena, V.K., Saxena, M., Ara, A., Pramod, A.B., Rajaram, M.L., Dorman, K.S., Majumdar, S. and Rasool, T.J. 2007. Molecular cloning and sequencing of MHC class II beta 1 domain of turkey reveals high sequence identity with chicken. International Journal of Immunogenetics 34, 97–105

Anand, S.K., Harpreet Singh and S.K.Pal. 1993. Level of bacterial load on guinea fowl fresh egg shell and internal content. Indian J. Poult. Sci. 28 :259-261.

Ansari, H.A. and Harpreet Singh. 1983. Kargology of guinea fowl *Numeda meleagria* Proceedings Xth Poultry Science Conference. IPSA. Madras AGB: 7-8.

Atul Gupta, M. K. Singh, S.K. Shukla, P.K. Shukla, H.N. Singh and Deepak Sharma 2008b. SSCP analysis for b1 domain of BLB 2 gene in guinea fowl and its association with antibody response to SRBC in guinea fowl., pp 202. In International Conference on "Current trends in Biotechnology & Implications in Agriculture" at SVP University of Agriculture & Technology, Meerut on 19th-21st Feb., 2009, pp 202.

Atul Gupta, M. K. Singh, Vinay Kumar, P.K. Shukla, H.N. Singh and Deepak Sharma 2008a. B haplotyping in guinea fowl using microsatellite based method. Pp 201. In International Conference on "Current trends in Biotechnology & Implications in Agriculture" at SVP University of Agriculture & Technology, Meerut on 19th-21st Feb., 2009, pp 202.

Avery, S., Rothwell, L., Degen, W.D., Schijns, V.E., Young, J., Kaufman, J. and Kaiser, P. 2004. Characterization of the first non-mammalian T2 cytokine gene cluster: the cluster contains functional single-copy genes for IL-3, IL-4, IL-13, and GM-CSF, a gene for IL-5 that appears to be a pseudogene and a gene encoding another cytokine like transcript, *KK34. J. Interferon Cytokine Res.* 24: 600-610.

Baverstock, P.R., M. Adams, R.W. Polkinghomes and M. Gelder. 1982. A sex linked enzyme in birds, Z-chromosome consevation but no dosage compensation. Nature 296:763-766.

Becker, W.A. 1986. *Manual of Quantitative Genetics.* Academic Enterprises, Pullman, Washington, D.C.

Belterman, R.H.R. and L.E.M. De Boer 1984. A kryological study of 55 species of birds, including karyotypes of 39 species new to cytology. Genetics 65: 39-68.

Bitgood, W.J. and R.N. Shoffner 1990. Cytology and Cytogenetics. In Crawford R.D. ed *Poultry Breeding and Genetics*. Elsevier Amsterdam. pp 401-428.

Bohren, B.B. 1975. Designing artificial selection experiments for specific objectives. *Genetics,* 80: 205-220.

Bourlet,Y., Behar,G., Guillemout,F., Frechin, N., Billault.A. and Chassee,A., 1988.Isolation of chicken major histocompatibility complex of class II B-L b chain sequences: comparison with mammalian beta chain and expression in lymphoid organs. EMBO Journal 7: 1031-1039

Briles ,W., McGibbon ,W. and Irwin, M. 1950. On multiple alleles affecting cellular antigens in the chicken. Genetics.35:633-640

Burt DW: Origin and evolution of avian minichromosomes. *Cytogenet Genome Res* 2002, 96:97-112.

Buschinelli, A. 1962. Experiments on vegetative hybridization in birds. World's Poultry Science Journal 18:246-254.

Caldwell, R.B. Kierzek, A.M. Arakawa, H. Bezzubov, Y. Zaim, J. Fiedler, P. Kutter, S. Blagodatski, A. Kostovska, D. Koter, M. Plachy, J. Carninci, P. Hayashizaki, Y. and Buerstedde, J.M. 2005. Full length cDNAs from chicken bursal lymphocytes to facilitate gene function analysis. *Genome Biol.* 6: 110-116.

Casuka, J. 1980. Polymorphism of guinea fowl egg white and the effect of denaturation factors on phenotypic manifestation. Proceedings. XVI International Conference of Animal Blood Biochemical Polymorphism Leningrad 4:75-80.

Croizeir, G. 1967. Etude de le transferrine des hybrids interspecifiques Gallus gallus x Numida meleagris. Annals Biologica Animal. Biochemistry and Biophysics 7:73-78.

Crowe, T.M. 1985. Guinea fowl. In Campbell B and E. Lack ed 1985. *A Dictionary of Birds.* Tr A.D. Poyser, Calton, Staffordshire.

De Boyer, L.E.M. 1984, New development vertibrate cytotaxonomy VIII . A current list of references on Avian Kryology Genetica 65:3-37.

Degen,W.G., Daal, N., Rothwell, L., Kaiser, P. and Schijns, V. E. 2005. Thl/Th2 polarization by viral and helminth infection in birds. *Vet. Microbiol.* 105: 163-167.

Delaney, M.E., Daniels, L.M., Swanberg, S.E., and Taylor, H.A. 2003. Telomeres in the chicken: Genome stability and chromosome ends. Poult. Sci. 82: 917–926.

Denisove, A and S.A. Khrustalev. 1974. The normal keryotype of the quinea fowl. Tsitologia Genetika 8:535- 539.

Dodgson, J.B., Cheng, H.H. and Okimoto, R. 1997. DNA marker technology: A revolution in animal genetics. Poultry Science. 76: 1108-1114.

Edwards, S.V., Hess, C.M., Gasper, J. and Garrigan, D. 1999. Towards an evolutionary genomics of the avian Mhc. Immunological Review. 167 : 119.

Epplen JT, Leipoldt M, Engel W, Schmidtke J: DNA sequence organization in avian genomes. Chromosoma 1978, 69:307-321.

Falconer, D.S. 1989. Introduction to Quantitative Genetics. Longman Group UK Ltd.Third edition.

G. Goyal, R.K.S. Bais, D. Sharma, S. Kumar and M.C. Kataria 2008a. Characterization and sequence analysis of Interferron gamma IFN-g gene of guinea fowl Numida meleagris. Abs No 36, pp 384. In IPSACON 08 on "Poultry Production in India : Threats and Opportunuties at Deptt of Poultry Science, College of Vety Sci & AH, Anand Agriculture University on 10th – 12th Dec., 2008.

G. Goyal, R.K.S. Bais, D. Sharma, S. Mehra and R.V. Singh 2008b.Genetic similarity and divergence for iNOS gene between guinea fowl and other poultry species. Abs No 41, pp 387. In IPSACON 08 on "Poultry Production in India : Threats and Opportunuties at Deptt of Poultry Science, College of Vety Sci & AH, Anand Agriculture University on 10th – 12th Dec., 2008.

Ghigi, A 1924. On the inheritance of colour in guinea fowl. Proc. 2nd World's Poultry Congress. Barcellona pp 18-19 loc. cit. Crawford 1998.

Ghigi, A, 1966. The breeding of guinea fowl in Italy. Proc. 13th World's Poultry Congress Kiev pp 137. loc. cit. Crawford 1998.Greenwood 1987

Goswami, S L. and Harpreet Singh. 1990. Macrochromosomal complement of indigenous guinea fowl. Indian Journal of Poultry Science 25:167-171.

Goswami, S.L. and Harpreet Singh. 1996 Chromosomal profile of guinea fowl, domestic fowl and hybrids Numigal. Indian Journal of Poultry Science 31:69-76.

Goto, R., Miyada ,C., Young ,S., Wallace ,R., Abplanalp ,H., Bloom ,S. and Brieles,W.E. 1988.Isolation of a cDNA clone from the B-G sub region of the chicken histocompatibility Bcomplex. Immunogenetics.102-109.

Greenwood, L. 1987. Mutations of guinea fowl. Poultry Press 20:15.

Gregory, T.R. 2002. A bird's-eye view of the C-value enigma: Genome size, cell size, and metabolic rate in the class Aves. Evolution 56: 121–130.

Guillemot, F., Billaut, A., Pourquie, O., Behar, A., Chasse, A. and Zoorob, R. 1988.A molecular map of the chicken major histocompatibility complex; The class II b genes are closely linked to the class I genes and the nucleolar organizer. EMBO.J. 7:2775-2785.

Hala, K., Palchy ,J. and Schulmannova ,J. 1981. Role of B- G antigen in the humoral immune response to the B- F antigen of chicken MHC. Immunogenetics, 14:393- 401.

Hazel, L. N., 1943. The genetic basis for constructing selection indices. *Genetics.* 28: 476-490.

Hilgert, I. and M. Voytiskova. 1959. Species heamoglobin in guinea fowl hen and domestic cock hybrids. Folia Biologica Praha 5:317-321.

Hosomichi,K., Shiina,T., Suzuki,S., Tanaka,M., Shimizu,S., Iwamoto,S., Hara,H., Yoshida,Y., Kulski,J.K., Inoko,H. and Hanzawa,K. 2006. The major histocompatibility complex MHC class IIB region has greater genomic structural flexibility and diversity in the quail than the chicken. BMC Genomics 7:322.

Jakowlew, S.B., Dillard, P.J., Sporn M.B and Roberts, A.B. 1988. Complementary deoxyribonucleic acid cloning of a messenger ribonucleic acid encoding transforming growth factor beta 4 from chicken embryo chondrocytes. *Mol. Endocrinol.* 2: 1186-1195.

Kaiser, P., Hester, M.W. and Rothwell, L. 1998. Structure of the chicken IFN-K gene and comparison to mammalian homologues. *Gene*. 207: 25–32.

Kaufman, J., Andersen, R., Avila, D., Engberg, J., Lambris, J., Salomonsen, J., Welinder, K. and Skjodi, K. 1992. Different features of the MHC class I hetrodimer have evolved at different rates. Chicken BF and beta 2-microglobulin sequences reveal invariant surface residues. J. Immunol., 148. 1532-1546.

Kaufman, J., Milne ,S., Gobel ,T.W.F., Walker ,R.A.1999 The chicken B locus is the minimal essential major histocompatibility complex. Nature 401:923-925.

Kierek-Jaszczuk, D. 1976. Electrophoretic forms of transferrins from blood, serum and egg contents of some selected species of poultry. Prace Materialy Zootechniczne 10:41-48.

Kindarle, D.D. 1994. Studies on the charactererisation, pathogenecity and immunogenicity of a field isolate of Newcastle disease virus from guinea fowl. M.V.Sc. Thesis; Deemed University, IVRI, Izatnagar.

Klein, J., Bontrop, R.E., Dawkins, R.L., Erlich, H.A., Gyllensten, U.B., Heise, E.R., Jones, P.P., Parham, P., Wakeland, E.K., Watkins, D.I. 1990. Nomenclature for the major hisocompatibility complex of different species: a proposal. Immunogenetics 31:217-219

Klein, S. and Ellendorff, F. 2000. Localization of *XhoI* repetitive sequences on autosomes in addition to the *W* chromosome in chickens and its relevance for sex diagnosis. *Anim. Genet.* 31: 104–109.

Kozi kova, L.V. 1984. Identification of sex chromosomes of guinea fowl. Cytology and genetics 18:75-77.

Kulski, J.K., Shiina, T., Anzai, T., Kohara, S. and Inoko, H. 2002 Comparative genomic analysis of the MHC: the evolution of class I duplication blocks, diversity and complexity from shark to man. Immunological Reviews. 190: 95.

Kumar S, Singh H and Sharma R D. 1997. Combining ability in guinea fowl broilers from a full diallel cross. Indian J. Animal Genetics & Breeding 191: 20-23.

Kumar, Sanjeev, Harpreet Singh and D.Sharma. 1995. Comparison of growth and conformation traits in three varities of guinea fowl. Indian.J. Poult. Sci.30:142-144.

Kumar, Sanjeev, Harpreet Singh and R.D. Sharma. 1997. Prediction of annual production on the basis of part record egg production in guinea fowl. Indian. J. Poult. Sci. 32: 122-125.

Lima-Rosa, C.A.V., Canal, C.W., Streck, A.F., Freitas, L.B., Delgado-Canedo, A., Bonatto, S.L. and Salzano et al. 2004. B-F DNA sequence variability in Brazilian blue egg Caipira chicken. Animal Genetics. 35 : 278-284.

Lin, A.W., Chang, C.C. and McCormick, C.C. 1996. Molecular cloning and expression of an avian macrophage nitric-oxide synthase cDNA and the analysis of the genomic 5′-flanking region. J. Biol. Chem. 271 20: 11911-11919.

Matzke, M.A., Varga, F., Berger, H., Schernthaner, J., Schweizer, D., Mayr, B., and Matzke, A.J.

1990. A 41–42 bp tandemly repeated sequence isolated from nuclear envelopes of chicken erythrocytes is located predominantly on microchromosomes. Chromosoma 99: 131–137.

Micek, J and V. Malik. Phylogenetic evolution of the K-factor. Sexlinked feathering rate in guinea fowl Nakamura et al. 1990 young and its practical use. Vedecke Prace Hydinarstovo 9:125-134.

Miller, H.C. & Lambert, D.M. 2004 Gene duplication and gene conversion in class II MHC genes of New Zealand robins Petroicidae. Immunogenetics, 56, 178.

Miller, M.M., Bacon, L.D., Hala, K., Hunt, H.D., Ewald, S.J., Kaufman, J., Zoorob, R., Briles ,W.E.2004. Nomenclature for the chicken major histocompatibility B and Y complex. Immunogenetics. 564:261-79.

Mishra, Sasmita. 1997. Studies on pathogenicity, strain differentiation and antigenic characterization of Newcastle disease virus isolated from different avian species. Ph.D. Thesis; Deemed University, IVRI., Izatnagar.

Mongin, P. and M. Plouzeau. 1984. Guinea fowl. Pp 322-324. In Masson, I:L ed 1984. *Evolution of Domesticated Animals.* Hutchinson, London.

Mosmann, T.R, Cherwinski, H., Bond, M.W., Giedlin, M.A. and Coffman, R.L. 1986. Two types of murine helper T cell clone. I. Definition according to' profiles of lymphokine activities and secreted proteins. J. Immunol. 136: 2348-2357.

Mosmann, T.R. and Coffman, R.L. 1989. TH1 and TH2 cells: different patterns of lymphokine secretion lead to different functional properties. Annu. Rev. Immunol. 7:145-173.

Mundra, B.L.1990. Inheritance of body weight and confirmation traits in guinea fowl *Numida Meleagris.* M.V.Sc Thesis, Submitted to Deemed University, IVRI, Izatnagar.

Mundra,B.L., K.L. Raheja and Harpreet Singh. 1993. Genetic and phenotypic parameter estimates for growth and conformation traits in guinea fowl. Indian J. Anim.Sci., 63:445-450.

Pal, S. K. and Harpreet Singh 1996b. Inhertance of erythrocytic glutthione concentration in guinea fowl. Indian Journal of Poultry Science 31:223-225.

Pal, S.K. and Harpreet Singh 1997a. Inhertance of wing feather development rate in guinea fowl Numida meleagris. British Poultry Science 38:245-248.

Pal, S.K. 1992. Genetic Characterisation of indigenous guinea fowl Numida meleagris germplasm. Ph.D. Thesis Deemed University, IVRI , Izatnagar.

Pal, S.K. and Harpreet Singh 1992. Protein polymorphism in guinea fowl. Proc. 19th World's Poultry Congress Sept. 19-24. 1992. Amsterdam. 3:367-370.

Singh, Harpreet and D.P. Singh 1988a. Studies on protein polymorphism in indigenous guinea fowl populations. Indian Journal of Poultry Science 23:66-71.

Pal, S.K. and Harpreet Singh 1997b. Inheritance of intera-erythrocytic potassium level variations in guinea fowl. Indian Journal of Poultry Science 32:292-295.

Pal, S.K. and Harpreet Singh. 1994 Pre - and post-embroyonic heamoglobin variations in guinea fowl. Indian Journal of Animal Science 64: 153-156.

Pal, S.K. and Harpreet Singh. 1996a. Genetic variation of guinea fowl alkaline phosphatase. Indian Journal of Poultry Science 31:101-105.

Panisup, A.S., Mohanty, G.C., Verma, K.C. and Singh, R. 1990. Occurrence of avian leukosis sarcoma group specific viral antigen in certain types and breeds of birds. Proc. 13th Poultry Science Conference & Symposium held by IPSA on 20th-22nd Dec., 1990 at Bombay. PMHE-17.

Pharr,G.T., Bacon,L.D. and Dodgson,J.B. 1993. Analysis of B-L betachain gene expression in two chicken cDNA libraries. Immunogenetics 37(5): 381-385.

Piccini, E and. Stella, 1970 Some avian karyotypes. Caryologia 23:189-702.

Pirchner, F., 1983. Population Genetics in Animal Breeding. Plenum Press, New York.

Rout, P.K. 1990. Genetics of retrovirus subgroup-A induced tumours in chorioallentoic membrane of embryos and in liver of chicks and guinea fowl species. M.V.Sc. Thesis; deemed University; IVRI, Izatnagar.

Sajjnar, C.M. 1994. Genetic studies on non-specific antimicrobial defenses of guinea fowl eggs. M.V.Sc. Thesis; Deemed University; IVRI, Izatnagar.

Satyendra Kumar, Jose Mathew, S. Mehra, S. K. Shukla and Deepak Sharma 2008. PCR-RFLP of BLB2 region in guinea fowl population diversified for immuno-competence and growth traits. Indian J. Poult. Sci. 43 : 139-142.

Saxena, V.K. 1993. Genetic studies on immuno-competence in guinea fowl numida meleagris. Ph.D. Thesis; Deemed University;IVRI, Izatnagar.

Saxena, V.K., D.K. Sharma, Harpreet Singh and S.C. Srivastava 1996. Acquired resistance against Argus persicus and its association with complement level in guinea fowl. J. Vety. Parasitology, 10: 191-195.

Schierman, L.W. and Nordskog, A.W. 1961. Relationship of blood type to histocompatibility in chickens. Science. 134:1008-1009.

Schmid M, Nanda L, Guttenbach M, Steinlein C, Hoehn M, Schartl M, Haaf T, Weigend S, Fries R, Buerstedde JM, Wimmers K, Burt DW, Smith J, A'Hara S, Law A, Griffin DK, Bunstead N, Kaufman J, Thomson PA, Burke T, Groenen MA, Crooijmans RP, Vignal A, Fillon V, Morisson M, Pitel F, Tixier-Boichard M, Ladjali-Mohammedi K, Hillel J, Maki-Tanila A, Cheng HH, Delany ME, Burnside J, Mizuno S: First report on chicken genes and chromosomes 2000. *Cytogenetics and Cell Genetics* 2000, 90:169-218.

Sharma Deepak .2009. Final Report of project "Genetic studies for guinea fowl improvement". Submitted to ICAR, New Delhi

Sharma Deepak 2007. Persistency of response to Sheep RBC in guinea fowl at different weeks of age. Indian J. Poultry Science 42: 331-332.

Sharma Deepak and Harpreet Singh 2005. Breeding Guinea fowl for improved performance. The Indian J Anim. Breeding & Genet. 26 1,2: 60-67.

Sharma Deepak, K.B.C. Appa Rao, H.P. Singh and S.M. Totey 1998. Random amplified polymorphic DNA RAPD for evaluating genetic relationship among guinea fowl varieties. Genetical Analysis : Biomolecular Engieneering 14 : 125-128.

Sharma Deepak, U.B.Singh, L.M.S. Nayal,Suneel Singh and R.V. Singh 2000 Carcass characteristics of improved guinea fowl at different weeks of age. Indian J. Poult. Sci. 352:224-225.

Sharma Deepak,, K.B.C. Appa Rao and A.K. Rawat 1999. Restriction enzyme analysis of satellite DNA components from poultry genome. Indian J. Animal Sciences 699 : 711-714.

Shiraishi, K. and Y. Hirai. 1983. Genetic Variants of liver and pancreas mannosephosphate isomerase in the Guinea fowl. Japanese Journal of Genetics 58:373-375.

Shiraishi, K., N. Iwase, T. Ishii and Y. Hirai. 1979. Blood groups and their gene frequencies in the guinea fowl. Japanese Poultry Science 16:93-99.

Shiraishi, K., S. Watanabe, T. Shibata and Y. Hirai. 1978. Genetic polymorphism of serum albumin and serum amylase in guinea fowl. Japanese Poultry Science 15:302-307.

Singh Harpreet, S.K. Pal and M.P. Mall. 1995. Identification of guinea fowl red cell membrane specificities with natural haemagglutinins. Indian Journal of Poultry Science 30:25-30.

Singh S. K., S. Mehra , Vinay Kumar , Sanjeev K. Shukla , A. Tiwari, G. Goyal , M. Mehra, Jose Mathew and Deepak Sharma 2010b. Sequence variability in the BLB2 region among guinea fowl and other poultry species International Journal of Genetics and Molecular Biology, Vol. 23, March, 2010

Singh S. K., S. Mehra, S.K. Shukla, Vinay Kumar, A. Tiwari, M. Mehra, Giriraj Goyal, Jose Mathew and Deepak Sharma 2010a. Nucleotide sequence variation in MHC class I region in guinea fowl. Accepted in International Journal of Poultry Science.

Singh S.K., J. Mathew, J. Gupta, S. Mehra, G. Goyal and D. Sharma 2010c. Molecular characterization of MHC class II region in guinea fowl. Accepted in British Poultry Science.

Singh, A, Gupta, J., Churchil, R.R., Sharma, D. and Singh, R.V. 2005. Genetic relatedness between red jungle fowl and other poultry species for BLB2 gene. Indian J Anim Genet. & Breeding. 26 : 18-20.

Singh, D.P., Harpreet Singh and Ram Gopal. 1989. Variation in feed consumption, feed efficiency and gain in body weight at different weeks of age in guinea fowl. Proc. Vth Natl. Seminar on Genetics Appl. Live. Prod. held Oct.21-23. 1989.; GUA, Anand, B.82.

Singh, Harpreet and B. Panda. 1984. Guinea fowl production status and its future in India. Poultry Guide. XXI (12): 39-43.

Singh, Harpreet and D.P. Singh. 1990. Genetic parameters of egg production and quality traits in indigenous guinea fowl. Proc. 13th Poult. Sci. Conf. & Symp. IPSA, held Dec. 20-22, 1990; Vety. College, Bombay. AGB-59: p. 32.

Singh, Harpreet, D.P.Singh and Gopal 1988a. Inheritance of body weights of guinea fowl. Indian J. Poult. Sci., 23:107-112.

Singh, Harpreet, P.S. Bedi, J. Kumari and R.D.Sharma, 1996. Genetic studies on immunocometence in guinea fowl. Proc.XX World's Poultry Congress, WPSA, held Sept. 2-8. New Delhi. Vol. 4: 510.

Singh, Harpreet, S.K. Pal and K.L.Raheja. 1993.Genetic and phenotypic parameters for egg production and egg quality traits in guinea fowl. Indian. J. Poult. Sci. 28:12-19.

Singh, Harpreet. 1998. Characterization and Evaluation of Indigenous Guinea fowl. Central Avian Research Institute, Izatnagar. 243 122 India.

Singh, S.K. 2008. Genetic polymorphism in BLB2 region and its association with immunocompetence and production traits in guinea fowl Numida meleagris. PhD thesis, Submitted to BU, Jhansi.

Singh,Harpreet, A.E.Nivasarkar C.L.Suman. 1991.Growth curve analysis and genetic parameters of body weight in indigenous guinea fowl. Indian J. Poult.Sci.,26:20-25.

Singh,Harpreet, D.P.Singh, and R.Gopal.1988b. Body measurements as crierion of growth in indigenous guinea fowl. India J.Anim.Prod., 20:37-44.

Snedecor, G. W. 1940 Statistical Methods Applied to Experiments in Agriculture and Biology. The Iowa State College Press, Ames, Iowa.

Somes, R.G. Jr. 1990. Mutations and major variants in guinea fowl. In Crawford, R.D. 1990 ed. *Poultry Breeding and Genetics*. Elsevier Amsterdam. pp 363-370.

Somes, R.G. Jr. 1992. Guinea fowl plumage colours. Personal communication.

Somes, R.G. Jr. 1996. Guinea fowl plumage color inheritance, with particular attention on dun color. Journal of Heredity 87: 138-142.

Srivastava, S.C. 1989. Feeding behavior of arugs persicus. Oken Acrina Argasidae on guinea fowl. Indian J. Parasitol. 13:237-238.

Srivastava, S.C. and Singh Harpret. 1988. Inherent tick resistance in guinea fowl: Preliminary obdervations. Procc. 12th Poultry Science Conference & Symposium held by IPSA on 8th-10th Dec., 1988 at CARI, Izatnagar. AGB: 62.

Stock, A.D. and T.D. Bunch. 1982. The evolutionary implications of chromosomes banding pattern homologies in the bird order Galliformes. Cytogenetics and Cell Genetics 34:136-148.

Takahashi, K. & Nei, M. 2000 Efficiencies of fast algorithms of phylogenetic inference under the criteria of maximum parsimony, minimum evolution and maximum likelihood when a large number of sequences are used. Molecular Biology and Evolution, 17, 1251.

Valenta, M. and A. Mikolasek. 1971. [Albumen polymorphism of guinea fowl eggs N. meleagaris. Sbormik Vysoke Skoly Zemedelske V Praze, Fakulta Agronomika. B. Zivocisna Vyroba. 113-123.

Vandergon, T.L. and Reitman, M. 1994. Evolution of chicken repeat 1 *CR1* elements: Evidence for ancient subfamilies and multiple progenitors. Mol. Biol. Evol. 11: 886–898.

Van-Hoeson, R. and L. Stromberg (ed.) 1975. *Guinea Fowl*. Strombery Publishing Co. Fort Dodge, Iowa Somes, R:G. Jr 1988.

Vijh, R.K., Sahai, R. and Singh, Harpreet. 1997. Cytogenetic studies on guinea fowl. Final Report. NBAGR. Karnal pp 1-10.

Wang, X., Li, J., and Leung, F.C. 2002. Partially inverted tandem repeat isolated from the pericentric region of chicken chromosome 8. *Chromosome Res.* 10: 73–82. Telomeres in the chicken: Genome stability and chromosome ends. Poult. Sci. 82: 917–926.

Wittzell,H., Bernot,A., Auffray,C. and Zoorob,R.1999. Concerted evolution of two Mhc class II B loci in pheasants and domestic chickens. Mol. Biol. Evol. 16 4: 479-90

Wood-Gush, D.G.M. 1985. Domestications. In Campbell, B and E. Lack T. & A.D. Poyser eds. Calton, Stafford shire.

Xia, C., Lin, C.Y., Xu, G.X., Hu, T.J. and Yang, T.Y. 2004. cDNA cloning and genomic structure of the duck Anas platyrhynchos MHC class I gene. Immunogenetics. 56 : 304-309.

Zeuner, F.E. 1963. A History of Domesticated Animals. Hutchinson London.

Zoorob, R., Behar, G., Kroemer, G. and Auffray, C., 1990.Organisation of a functional chicken class II gene. Immunogenetics 31:179-187.

Zoorob, R., Bernot, A., Renoir, A.D.M., Choukri, F. and Auffray, C. 1993. Chicken MHC class II b genes, analysis of interallelic and intralocus sequence variance. Eur. J. Immunol. 23: 1139-1195.

❑❑❑